# The Ketogenic Solution for Lymphatic Disorders

## Lose Weight and Dramatically Reduce Lymphatic Swelling

### Leslyn Keith

Gutsy Badger
YORK,

## Copyright © 2019 Leslyn Keith

All rights reserved. No part of this book may be reproduced, distributed or transmitted in any form or by any means, including photocopying, recording, or other electronic or mechanical methods, without the prior written permission of the publisher, except in the case of brief quotations embodied in critical reviews and certain other noncommercial uses permitted by copyright law. For permission requests, write to the author at the email address below.

Leslyn Keith, OTD, OTR/L, CLT-LANA
leslynkeithot@gmail.com
leslynkeith.com

All of the information provided in and throughout this Publication is intended solely for general information and should NOT be relied upon for any particular diagnosis, treatment or care. This is not a substitute for medical advice or treatment. This Publication is only for general informational purposes. It is strongly encouraged that individuals and their families consult with qualified medical professionals for treatment and related advice on individual cases before beginning any diet. Decisions relating to the prevention, detection and treatment of all health issues should be made only after discussing the risks and benefits with your health-care provider, taking into account your personal medical history, your current situation and your future health risks and concerns. If you are pregnant, nursing, diabetic, on medication, have a medical condition, or are beginning a health or weight control program, consult your physician before using products or services discussed in this Publication and before making any other dietary changes. The author and publisher cannot guarantee that the information in this Publication is safe and proper for every reader. For this reason, this Publication is sold without warranties or guarantees of any kind, express or implied, and the author and publisher disclaim any liability, loss or damage caused by the contents, either directly or consequentially. Statements made in this Publication have not been evaluated by the U.S. Food and Drug Administration or any other government regulatory body. Products, services and methods discussed in this Publication are not intended to diagnose, treat, cure or prevent any disease.

*The Ketogenic Solution for Lymphatic Disorders* / Leslyn Keith

ISBN-13: 978-1-943721-12-2 (Paperback)
ISBN-13: 978-1-943721-11-5 (Electronic)

# Dedication

*This book is dedicated to my patients and their families, and to the lymphedema therapy community. I hope this book helps you help others.*

# Contents

*Dedication* .................................................................................. 3
*Acknowledgements* ..................................................................... 9
*Introduction* ............................................................................. 11

**Chapter 1   Does This Lymph Make Me Look Fat?** ........................ 17

    Lymphatic Disorders ............................................................. 17
    Lymphedema ......................................................................... 17
    Lipedema ............................................................................... 19
    Edema .................................................................................... 20
    Other Lymphatic Disorders .................................................. 20
    Function of the Lymphatic System ....................................... 21
    The Special Role of Adipose Tissue ...................................... 23
    Adipose Tissue and the Lymph System: Function at the Junction. 26
    Fat Proliferation with Lymph Stasis ..................................... 27
    Obesity-Induced Lymphedema ............................................. 28

**Chapter 2   Weight of Evidence** ................................................... 31

    Losing Weight ....................................................................... 31
    What Doesn't Work .............................................................. 34

## Chapter 3  How Dietary Fat Will Save the Day ............................................. 41

Ketogenic Diet for Health and Weight Loss ................................................. 41
Ketogenic Diet for Lymphedema .................................................................. 50
Keto-Lymphedema Study 2017 ..................................................................... 52
Ketogenic Diet for Lipedema ......................................................................... 56

## Chapter 4  A Ketogenic Way of Eating Impacts More Than Just Weight ...... 61

Cancer, Obesity and Lymphedema ................................................................ 62
Bariatric Surgery ............................................................................................. 65
Liposuction ...................................................................................................... 70
Gallstones and Cholecystectomy .................................................................. 71
Metabolic Syndrome ...................................................................................... 73
Lymphatics/Salt Connection ......................................................................... 77
The Malnutrition and Edema Connection .................................................. 81

## Chapter 5  How Keto Can Change Your Practice ......................................... 87

Scope of Practice: Can I Do That? ................................................................ 87
The Power of Group Intervention ................................................................ 91
Addressing Weight Issues with Clients ........................................................ 93
Individual Weight Management Counseling .............................................. 96

## Chapter 6  Regarding Opposition ................................................................ 101

Sez Who? ........................................................................................................ 101
Fat Phobia ...................................................................................................... 104

## Chapter 7  Ketogenic Nutrition Guide ........................................................ 111

How Strict Does One Need to Be? .............................................................. 115

## Appendix I  Ketogenic Ingredients ............................................................. 117

Ketogenic Shopping List .............................................................................. 119

## Appendix II  Resources ..................................................................... 121

Lymphatic Therapy ........................................................... 121
Workshops ......................................................................... 121
Health Websites ................................................................ 122
Food Log Websites............................................................ 122
Low-Carb Health Providers ........................................... 123
Videos................................................................................. 123
Social Media ...................................................................... 124
Books................................................................................... 124

## Appendix III  Lymphatic Lifestyle Solutions Program ..................... 127

## References ........................................................................................ 131

## About the Author ............................................................................ 141

# Acknowledgements

I would like to acknowledge the influence and support from the following people: Karen Ashforth, Rose Marie Battaglia, Kelly Bell, Lesli Bell, Shoosh Crotzer, Ellen Davis, Esteban Delgado, Ron and Melody DeMoss, Guenter Klose, Katrina Harris, Maureen McBeth, Jean Radin, Lorie Richards, Bill Robinson, JoAnn Rovig, Carol Rowsemitt, Catherine Seo, Eric Westman, and Jay Wortman.

In addition, thank you to all of the women who are involved with the Beyond Lipedema MasterClass, Lipedema & Keto WOE Dream Team and Keto Lipedema Facebook groups; all of the participants who were part of my research; and all those who were willing to take a chance on changing to a keto lifestyle.

# Introduction

Spending time in any public place, such as an airport or shopping center, one can see myriad examples of people with obesity and weight-related lymphedema. Overweight women in short sleeve tops might display a distinctive shelf pattern at their elbows or have forearms that come to an abruptly narrower wrist. Often, a man can be seen in shorts with the telltale hemosiderin staining to his lower calves, suggesting chronic venous insufficiency, or have a distended abdomen riding over his belt. Some of these presentations can look quite painful.

Overweight and obesity commonly travel cheek by jowl with symptoms of lymphedema. The purpose of this book is to explain why this is so and to help doctors and therapists to understand that a lymphatic disorder cannot be treated if one of its major comorbidities or possible underlying causes remains unaddressed. In addition, I will show why conventional treatments have not alleviated the epidemic of obesity that people in this country and most of the world are experiencing and suggest a better option for management using a ketogenic diet.

Presently, it is more likely than not for a client who is referred to a clinical practice for lymphedema therapy to also have a severe weight problem. Using conventional treatment tools and protocols which tend to deal with only the swelling, successful outcomes seemed to be dwindling. In workshops and roundtable discussions which I have moderated at lymphedema conferences over the past few years on the topic of obesity and lymphedema, the majority of therapists have reported a trend

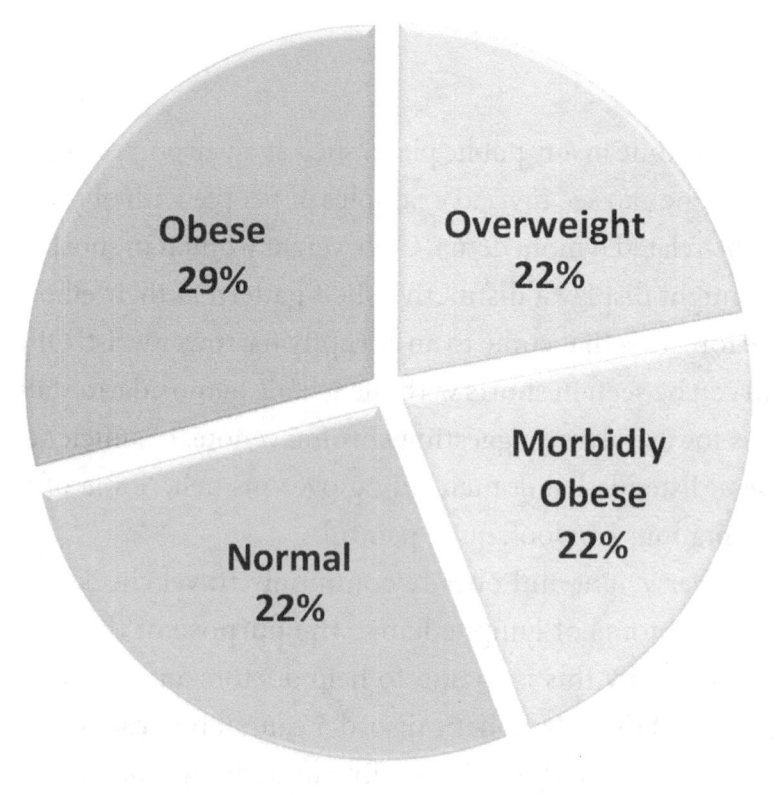

*Figure 1. Distribution of patients by Body Mass Index (BMI). Three quarters of my patients during a six month period were overweight or obese.*

of increasing obesity among their clientele. These lymphedema therapists report that now well over 50% of their clients are obese, with a large portion of those being morbidly obese. I was not surprised when I found this trend reflected in my own clinic. Many eager interns have volunteered in my clinic, and I gave one the exercise of quantifying the percentage of my clients that were overweight or obese. Figure 1 shows the Body Mass Index (BMI) distribution of patients seen during a six month time period in 2014 in my practice.

An increasing number of lymphedema therapy clinics are mandating that their obese clients with lymphedema must be involved in a weight loss program concomitantly with their lymphedema treatment.[1,2] My clinic is also instituting this requirement, as successful treatment of clients with both lymphedema and obesity is virtually impossible if weight management is ignored. Obese clients often return for treatment year after year with no permanent beneficial outcomes. The salient point of this book is to convince medical personnel dealing with clients with lymphedema to pay as much attention to their clients' obesity as to the lymphedema itself.

A few years ago I became interested in weight loss strategies which differ from conventional approaches. These effective methods, although neither new nor unique, had been hidden in a dietary milieu dominated by conventional wisdom represented by the USDA's food pyramid and more recently, MyPlate.[3] In discussions with my overweight clients, I came to the conclusion that they were, in fact, trying to follow their doctor's, and thus the government's, recommendations in their efforts to lose weight. Sadly, many had failed time and again to lose their excess body fat, or to keep it off, had they managed to achieve any weight loss at all. Many, if not most, had taken the failure as their own. At the time that they were referred to me, both patient and doctor had, in effect, given up on solving their weight condition.

My strategy had to be different.

One of my clients gave me Gary Taubes' *Why We Get Fat, and What to Do About It*. The book sat on a shelf for a few days until my partner Bill picked it up and read it. He went on to read Taubes' *Good Calories, Bad Calories*, and became inspired to amass shelves full of books on the subject of nutrition related to weight loss and energy partitioning. His enthusiastic exclamations while reading enticed me and I ended up reading extensively on the subject as well. I have now collected a great number of books and studies which bolster the idea that weight loss and maintenance are more affected by a diet's macronutrient content than by limits on calories. These ideas will be discussed in Chapter 3.

In the years since, I have expanded my typical consultation with my clients to include proper weight management technique as an adjunct to conventional treatment of their lymphedema and, consequently, the number of successful outcomes among my clients with obesity has been rising. The rationale for focusing on weight loss in addition to established lymphedema therapy protocol is based on the fact that adipose tissue is not just idle tissue, but interacts hormonally with all other systems in the body. Of particular importance to the topic here is the interaction between lymphatics and adipose tissue. Adipose cells were, until recently, seen as only repositories of fat which did not interact with other systems. That view has changed, and evidence now clearly demonstrates that adipose cells communicate through the release of hormones, causing multiple reactions in the body (see Chapter 1).

Further study has revealed to me that lymphatic and adipose tissues work quite closely together and any change in one is reflected quickly in a response in the other. This is typical of hundreds of other feedback mechanisms in the body.[4] Isolating one thing on which to focus when treating any disease is shortsighted. This has solidified in my mind the concept that to effectively deal with a client's lymphedema, the clinician must address any excess weight of the client along with their lymphedema. A scientific approach needs to be utilized when incorporating any treatment method and the science has come down on the side of ketogenic nutrition for weight loss as being the most effective and healthiest approach.[5-8] Unfortunately, the utilization of this way of eating for weight loss has mainly been limited by a fear of fat consumption.

Fat phobia in relation to lymphedema treatment is remarkable when considered in light of the fact that the lymphatic system runs substantially on lipids and is the major transporter of dietary fat into blood circulation. The latest release of Dietary Guidelines for Americans now concedes that dietary fats, including cholesterol and saturated fat, are no longer the villains they were portrayed to be over the past half century.[9]

It has been a joy to watch clients, who had a lack of success on prior weight loss programs, use the methods I recommend. They reduce their weight, take a load of pressure off their swelling and increase the functionality and health of their body. In several cases, simply losing weight has caused clients' lymphedema to spontaneously reduce. I'm gratified when a client comes back months or years later to thank me for showing them how it all fits together and for giving them the information and the ability to resolve their swelling.

This information has been available for many decades, yet few practitioners are putting it into practice. One of my goals for writing this book is to increase the understanding of the relationship between lymphatic disorders and obesity among medical professionals. When clinicians are armed with this knowledge, they will be better able to assist in lessening their clients' suffering. Using this knowledge, along with a complete program that I have developed to introduce and guide clients to ketogenic nutrition (a lifestyle modification course called *Lymphatic Lifestyle Solutions*–see Appendix III), clinicians will be more successful in their therapy practices. My wish is that more therapists will experience clients returning to their lymphedema clinics, not for more treatment, but to give thanks for introducing them to this healthy lifestyle and the better management of their lymphedema.

# Chapter 1

# Does This Lymph Make Me Look Fat?

## Lymphatic Disorders

### Lymphedema

Lymphedema is fluid retention in tissues that presents as swelling of a body part. According to the International Society of Lymphology Consensus Document,[10] an accurate diagnosis of lymphedema is only made when edema results from an impairment of the lymphatic system causing a reduced transport capacity. Edema that occurs in an intact lymphatic system that is overwhelmed by an increased fluid load will be addressed separately.

The most common etiology of lymphedema worldwide is filariasis, a parasitic infection that damages the lymphatics and is primarily limited to tropical and subtropical regions. Poor access

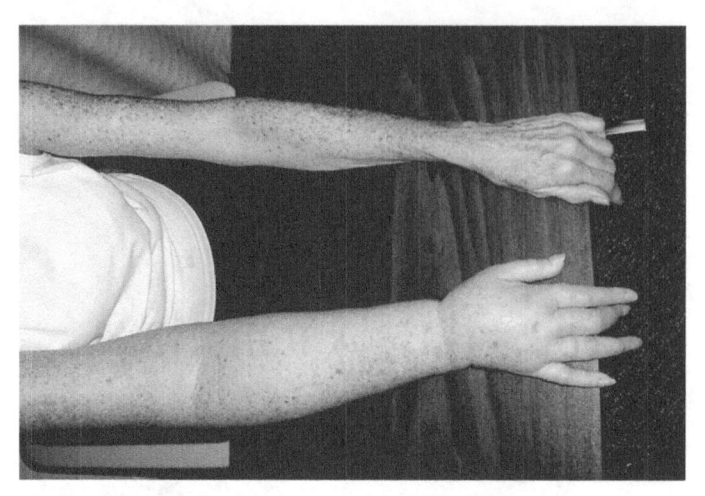

*Figure 2. Breast cancer treatment-related lymphedema*

to health care, limited education regarding transmission prevention, improper hygiene and skin care contribute to increased incidence. In the United States, however, more common reasons for the development of lymphedema are surgery, especially for cancer when lymph nodes are removed, radiation treatments, and congenital malformation of the lymphatics. These all can result in a disruption of lymphatic drainage that leads to swelling in the affected body region.

Conservative treatment of lymphedema has evolved to consist of manual lymph drainage (a gentle massage technique that reroutes fluid around obstructions), compression bandaging, decongestive exercises, meticulous skin care, and compression garments. Other modalities which may be employed to augment management of lymphedema can include microsurgery and the use of pneumatic compression pumps. Recently, people with lymphedema, as well as clinicians and researchers, are investigating the importance of nutrition in improving lymphedema treatment outcomes.

# Lipedema

Lipedema is generally described as a chronic and generally progressive adipose tissue disorder that almost exclusively affects women. It is characterized by a symmetrical enlargement of the lower body due to excessive fatty deposits from waist to ankles, easy bruising, orthostatic edema, and pain. Onset seems to coincide with times of significant hormonal upheaval, such as during puberty, pregnancy and menopause.[11] Besides the disproportion between upper and lower body that occurs with lipedema, the most devastating feature may be that it is generally believed to be non-responsive to diet and exercise. First reported by physicians at the Mayo Clinic in 1940,[12] this condition continues to remain a poorly understood, largely underdiagnosed, and profoundly impactful syndrome.

Gender is a major determinant of adipose tissue distribution. Research has shown that in general men are more prone to lipolysis, or fat burning, and women tend more toward lipogenesis, or fat creation and storage.[13] Additionally, women have a tendency toward upper body lipolysis and lower body lipogenesis which

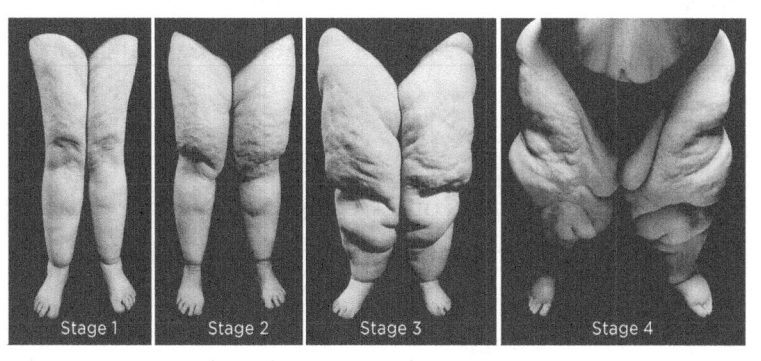

*Figure 3. Women with lipedema ranging from mild to severe. (The Lipedema Project. 2015-2019. All rights reserved. Used with permission.)*

may result in a lipedema presentation. During puberty, females increasingly store subcutaneous fat throughout the body, with concentrations at the hips, buttocks and thighs. Women tend also to be more sensitive to insulin, the fat storage hormone, which puts them at higher risk for weight gain than men.[14]

Although considered by some clinicians to not be a lymphatic disorder, lipedema is a condition of concern in this book because disrupted lymphatics are often a constituent of the condition. For instance, most women with this condition have some mild swelling and a significant number go on to also develop lymphedema.

## Edema

Swelling can also occur when the lymphatic system is intact but is completely overwhelmed with an excessive amount of fluid. When fluid overload is the origin of swelling rather than some mechanical insufficiency or obstruction, the term *edema* is used. Edema can result from organ failure (such as heart, kidney, or liver impairment), nutritional deficiency (which may occur due to malnutrition or bariatric surgery), injury or trauma (such as a broken bone or surgery), or as a side effect to a medication.

## Other Lymphatic Disorders

The following list provides other lymphatic disorders that tend to be more rare than lymphedema, lipedema and edema.

- Lymphangioma
- Lymphangiomatosis
- Gorham's Disease

- Lymphangiectasia
- Lymphangioleiomyomatosis
- Microcystic Lymphatic Malformation
- Hennekam Syndrome
- Waldmann Disease

## Function of the Lymphatic System

In the human body, the lymphatic system is equally as extensive as the cardiovascular system. Wherever there is a blood vessel, there is a corresponding lymph vessel. The importance of a well-functioning lymphatic system cannot be overstated, but this subject has unfortunately been little studied and largely ignored by medical research.[15] This vital system may be overlooked partly because, except for the milky-colored chyle in the gut, it is a transparent system of vessels that are hard to see with the naked eye. The three main functions of the lymphatic system are:

1. Immune surveillance
2. Fluid balance by the return of protein and water back to blood circulation
3. Fat transport from the gut into blood circulation

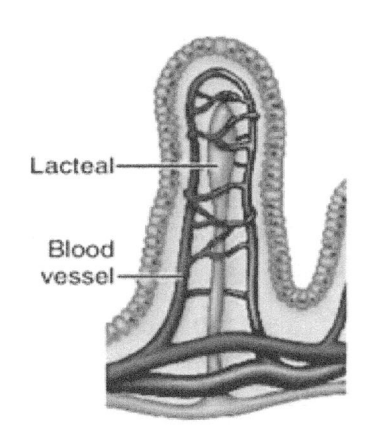

*Figure 4. Intestinal villi with blood and lymphatic vessels. The lymphatic lacteal is responsible for absorbing and transporting dietary fat.*

One of the most studied roles of the lymphatic system is its participation in immune surveillance, most often in the context of cancer. Lymphocytes, used to fight infection and promote immunity, are a major component of this patrol responsibility. Lymphocytes are stored in lymph nodes and the spleen, and can be deployed where needed.[16] Cancer metastasis is usually checked by sampling and examining regional lymph nodes. Removal of lymph nodes may impair immune functions to such a degree that some people with cancer-related lymphedema suffer repeated infections to the affected region.[17] We will see in the next chapter how the immune functions of the lymphatic system are powered by fatty acids.

The lymphatic system is essential to the maintenance of the body's fluid balance through its transport of water and macromolecules such as protein from the interstitium back to blood circulation. Once thought to act only as a backup to the venous system, the recent update of Starling's Equilibrium demonstrates that in reality the return of interstitial fluid to blood circulation is accomplished completely by the lymphatic system.[18]

The lymphatic system is responsible for transporting all dietary fat, with the exception of medium chain triglycerides, from the intestines to blood circulation. If the lymphatic system has been mostly disregarded by medical science, the significance of its job of transporting fat has been virtually invisible. Even lymphologists and lymphedema experts lump this responsibility of the lymphatic system together with removal of "waste material".[19] In fact, dietary fat is so important to our bodies that we have a system just for conveying that fat to where it is needed. Intestinal lymphatics, called lacteals, absorb dietary fat from the intestinal villi and deliver it to the thoracic duct, where it is then transported to the blood circulatory system via the subclavian vein.

## The Special Role of Adipose Tissue

An adequate amount of adipose tissue is essential for health. A disorder of too little fat (lipodystrophy) can place the individual at considerable metabolic risk.[20] Beyond the more obvious duties of adipose tissue such as mechanically cushioning delicate organs such as the eye, passively insulating the body, and storing energy, the endocrine function of adipose tissue is perhaps its most important work. Adipose tissue supplies energy and raw materials for the creation of hormones necessary for the proper operation of the whole body.

In only the last few decades has adipose tissue been considered to be an important endocrine organ in the human body. Its complexity has only recently been revealed through research which shows that adipose cells communicate with and influence virtually every other cell in the body. As the prejudice evoked by the word "fat" is dropped by researchers, more useful information about adipose tissue has created a new understanding of its important functions.

One adipose tissue-derived hormone of particular importance to our discussion is adiponectin. This adipokine is essential to lymphatic vasculature health due to its role in promoting vessel integrity.[21,22] Additionally, adiponectin has been shown to be insulin-sensitizing. Because the expression of adiponectin is suppressed in the presence of obesity, it is no surprise that the obese person becomes insulin resistant and develops leaky lymphatic vessels.

Fat tissue has recently been found to be an excellent source of stem cells, particularly from adipocytes found in the omentum. For this reason, plastic surgeons performing microsurgery for the treatment of lymphedema prefer to harvest lymph nodes for transfer from this stem cell-rich area in abdominal fat.[23]

Another significant role of adipose tissue is its ability to take in excess energy in the form of lipids which are then stored in adipocytes as triglycerides. In a healthy system, these stored lipids can be released as energy needs increase, as a means of buffering against reduced energy consumption.

Adipose tissue has the ability to absorb lipids and expand through two mechanisms: hyperplasia, the increase in the number of cells, and hypertrophy, the increase in size of those cells. Although an unhealthy state can be created by either method if a certain threshold is exceeded, hyperplasia is generally thought of as a better option than hypertrophy.[24] If hyperplasia has been accompanied with a healthy vascularization, ingress and egress of lipids in response to energy demands may be quite facile. With hypertrophy, vascularization is more likely to be compromised and the individual adipocytes can reach a size where they cannot take in any more lipids. This scenario causes the reduction of lipid transport into and out of adipocytes. A lessened ability of adipocytes to take in lipids results in an increased chance that the bloodstream will contain higher (unhealthful) levels of lipids in the form of triglycerides.[24]

Adipose tissue is not just one monolithic thing. Fat interacts with its surroundings and secretes hormones differently according to its location and composition. We now differentiate between brown, white, and more recently, beige adipose tissue. Brown adipose tissue, for instance, is much more metabolically active than other forms of fat and can generate its own heat by burning some of its stored lipids. White adipose tissue functions mainly as energy storage, and beige combines the two functions.[25]

Generally speaking, subcutaneous fat is considered to be beneficial, whereas visceral fat is recognized as troublesome. This had been thought to be simply a matter of pressure on internal organs. Although the mechanical occlusion of organ function plays a role, recent research has shown that adipose tissue in these disparate places secrete different adipokines which act in diverse ways. Even when adipose tissue from different areas of the body are experimentally isolated, they continue to express the same types of hormones they had been expressing in vivo.[26]

So, too, does the influence of adipose tissue change as the host's weight status changes. Adipose tissue acts as a repository of immune cells which have been created by the lymphatic system. A lean person's adipose tissue will harbor a different type of macrophage than will the adipose tissue of an individual with obesity.[27] Macrophages in adipose tissue of someone with obesity tend to be of a proinflammatory variety[26] further contributing to dysfunction and metabolic dysregulation.

Adipose tissue is a dynamic system, reacting to many varied inputs, worthy of a discussion much beyond the scope of this book. I encourage you to further study this important endocrine organ.

# Adipose Tissue and the Lymph System: Function at the Junction

In a healthy body, adipose tissue works closely with the lymphatic system. Invariably, lymph nodes are encased in a pad of adipose tissue. This is seen consistently in both the lean and the obese. One reason for the intimate relationship between adipose tissue and lymphatics is that the crucial work of the lymphatic system, namely its immunological functions, requires a ready source of energy. It has been well established that the lymphatic system is powered by fatty acids. Necessarily, acute inflammation will result in increased lipolysis in order to meet increased energy needs, while the consequence of a chronic inflammatory condition is adipocyte proliferation.[28,29]

Communication between adipose tissue and lymphatics is also apparent when obesity is present. Fat tissue becomes distressed when present in excessive amounts, and will signal the lymphatic system for immunological support. Lymphatics in turn, in the form of macrophages, signal inflammatory agents (such as TNF-alpha) in response to adipose tissue disturbance. A pathology, such as type 2 diabetes, can cause lymphatic vessels to become inefficient and leaky.[30] Professor Etelka Földi, MD, one of the pioneers of modern lymphology, has stated that insulin resistance can increase lymphatic load.[31] This demonstrates how lymphatic dysfunction can play a part in metabolic diseases such as obesity.

# Fat Proliferation with Lymph Stasis

*Links between lymphatic disorders and obesity*

Fascinating research into the intimate relationship between the lymphatic system and adipose tissue has occurred over the last decade. The role of the lymphatic system with lipid metabolism is far more complex and much more integral to human health than was previously thought. Recent research shows that adipose tissue function is an active process, rather than the previously characterized passive one. Dysfunctional or diseased body fat may play an important role in inflammation, diabetes, and obesity.[32] For instance, lymphedema therapists have long been aware of the propensity of a swollen limb to accumulate fat,[33] as well as a seemingly common association between hereditary lymphedema in the legs and obesity.[34] Why would this be so?

A very interesting cooperative relationship exists between the lymphatic system and adipose tissue to enable immune function. Several researchers have noted that lymphatic structures and fat tissue are usually found in very close proximity.[35,36] The lymphatic system has a preference for fatty acids as its fuel substrate. Immune functions can be carried out much more effectively if a ready energy source is nearby. It is theorized that the lymphatic system releases an agent that breaks down fatty reserves into fatty acids for use during an immune emergency and can replenish its supply of fuel by releasing another agent to cause fat tissue to proliferate.

Unfortunately, the chronic inflammation present with lymphedema sends an alert to the lymphatic system to stimulate the buildup of fat in the swollen limb. Long term presence of swelling suggests to the body a need for an immune response, so adipose tissue is encouraged to proliferate to provide a long term source of energy.[28] As it continues to expand, further dysfunction in the fat tissue develops. Both lymphatic and blood vessels become leaky, contributing to faulty circulation of nutrition and waste products to and from the cells, ineffective lymph drainage, and ultimately more swelling. Increased edema signals further immunological need which brings about further fat generation to meet energy needs.[35,37] And so the cycle between fat buildup in the limb and lymphedema persists.

## Obesity-Induced Lymphedema

Commonly, swelling can be caused merely by excess weight or obesity, termed obesity-induced lymphedema. The mechanism can be overt, such as in the case of a large panniculus where tissue can hang down from the waist and rest against the inguinal lymph nodes, creating a mechanical blockage. Likewise, venous hypertension, chronic venous insufficiency, and distended varicose veins can prevent efficient removal of fluid and are easily discernible by appearance. Clinical findings are typically reinforced by diagnostic tests, such as a venous Doppler.

Other mechanisms for obesity-induced lymphedema may be less obvious. The person with obesity is particularly vulnerable to being caught up in the cycle of adipose expansion and lymphedema, especially those with abdominal obesity. The abdomen has the greatest concentration of lymph nodes in the body and, as elsewhere in the body, the abdominal lymphatics are surrounded by a certain amount of healthy subcutaneous fat.

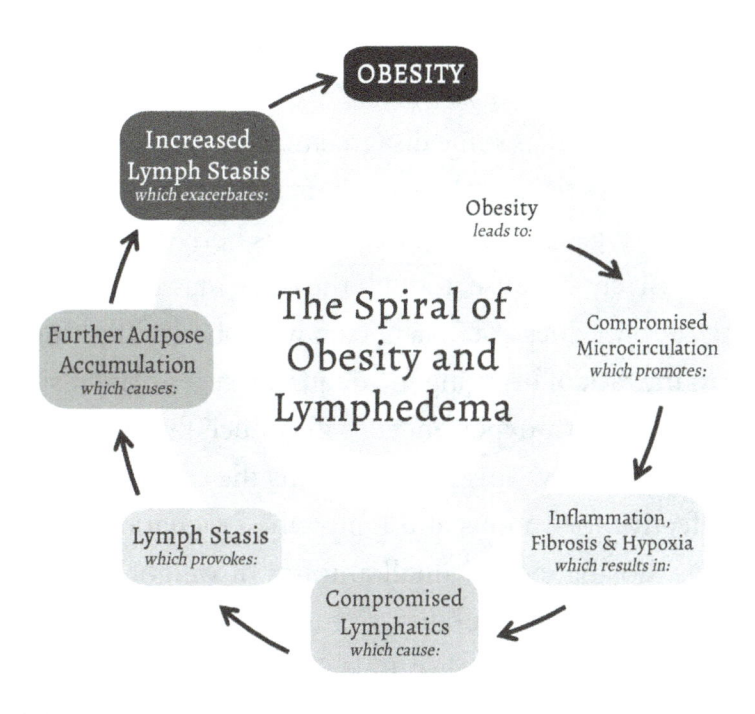

*Figure 5. The Spiral of Obesity and Lymphedema. The compromised microcirculation in excessive adipose tissue leads to hypoxia, fibrosis, and the expression of pro-inflammatory agents that harm lymphatic vessels. This creates more edema, which in turn encourages adipose tissue proliferation.*

When abdominal fat becomes overly excessive, proinflammatory agents, such as C-reactive protein, are not removed and thus contribute to further inflammation.[38] As discussed earlier, fat tissue expansion also suppresses the release of anti-inflammatory agents, such as adiponectin, needed to maintain lymphatic vessel health. Fortunately, with weight loss, adiponectin levels are re-established and there can be improvement in lymphatic function. When metabolic syndrome is a comorbidity of obesity, the body begins storing fat around organs such as the kidneys and liver. Ectopic fat impairs the function of these organs, causing even more limb swelling to develop.[39]

Although there is some disagreement among researchers,[40] stress on adipose tissue may also be increased with hypoxia, or inadequate oxygen, to adipocytes. Excess body mass taxes the lungs excessively, because, though the body may double in size, the lung capacity does not. In a person with obesity, the lungs are not up to the task of bringing in adequate oxygen. The resultant shortness of breath experienced will induce fatigue and lead to decreased activity. This in turn means the calf muscle pump is less effective for venous and lymphatic evacuation from the lower legs. Losing even a small amount of weight commonly results in much better mobility, restoring oxygen to the tissues and rejuvenating the muscle pump.

Regrettably, unless the cause of increased fluid load placed on a limb by obesity-induced lymphedema is addressed, a never ending battle will commence. It has been no surprise that patients with obesity have the least success in long-term management of their lymphedema. Obesity has a host of related conditions, such as cardiovascular disease, hypertension, reflux, sleep apnea, diabetes, arthritis, and some types of cancer. As with obesity and lymphedema, several of these additional disorders can also interact with lymphedema to exacerbate the overall unfavorable health of the client, and preclude the favorable outcome of treatment.

# Chapter 2

# Weight of Evidence

## Losing Weight

*"I had always been conscientious about eating according to the information I was given by my doctors over the years, but I gained weight no matter what I did."*

~John J., *Lymphatic Lifestyle Solutions* Participant

Now that the therapist understands the issue of weight being related to lymphedema, what is the preferred treatment to reduce the excess weight? There are as many ways to deal with weight issues as there are doctors and therapists. Also, different clients will respond to different approaches. What has become crystal clear over the past half century is that the conventional wisdom on weight loss has failed. Let me say that again. The people with weight problems have not failed. The conventional wisdom has failed.

What is the conventional wisdom on weight loss and how did it come to take its preeminent position? Through a series of inept science, bad studies, huge egos, political expediency and an unholy alliance between large food conglomerates, pharmaceutical companies and government, our institutions have disseminated the incorrect belief that achieving weight loss is always an equation of simple energy balance: a matter of eating less and moving more. The background on this history is beyond the purview of this book but readers may want to read more about this idea, which is well documented in *Good Calories, Bad Calories*, by Gary Taubes and *The Big Fat Surprise*, by Nina Teicholz.

The typical strategy for promoting weight loss over the last thirty to forty years has been to achieve a negative energy balance by eating less, exercising more, or both. This was initially promoted pervasively through the official publication of the Dietary Goals for the United States in 1977 that resulted in the USDA Food Pyramid.[41] Documentation of the prevalence of obesity in America demonstrates that the beginnings of the obesity epidemic occurred in the mid-1980s.[42] This epidemic has coincided with our government's recommendation to eat more carbohydrates, less fat and fewer total calories, and to exercise more.[43]

Weight loss programs abound. How can a person choose among the hundreds of books found in a typical bookstore promising easy weight loss? In addition, if they peruse Amazon or the many other online book dealers, the number of diet books available totals in the thousands. When that person goes to a medical practitioner, how can they be sure that they will get proper information? What can therapists do to make sure they are setting forth a useful method for weight loss?

Medical doctors and therapists are burdened with the responsibility of keeping current on information regarding their fields of practice. Research today is greatly facilitated by the internet. Any therapist connected to a teaching hospital should

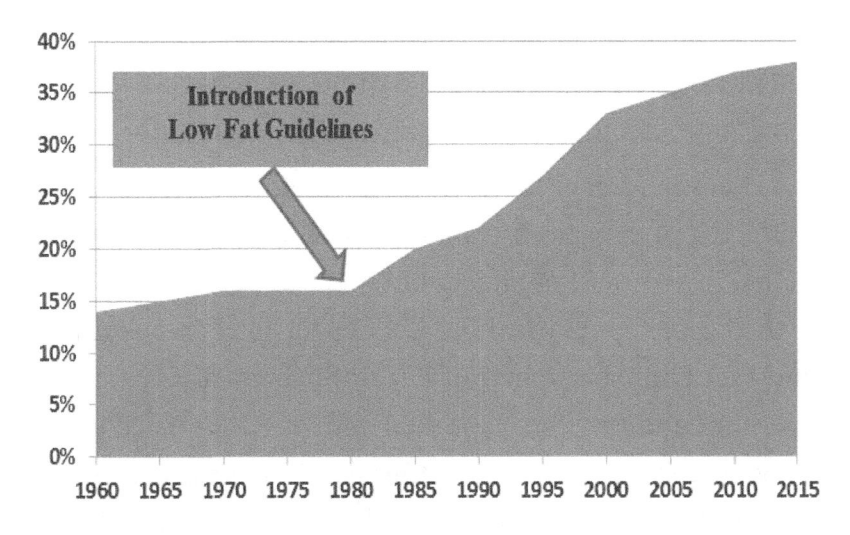

*Figure 6. The steep rise in US adults with obesity coincides with the introduction of Dietary Guidelines that recommended curtailing the intake of fat.*

have near immediate access to research papers they can download and examine themselves. It is important for medical professionals to scrutinize papers in their entirety, not just media reports of studies. Reading another author's conclusions, or a news report based on a press release leads to misinterpreted and misrepresented facts. Rather, by having access to the original peer reviewed article, or even by contacting the author, a better understanding of the research can be reached. The following section will discuss what we have traditionally done for weight management and why it doesn't work.

# What Doesn't Work

*How many diets have I been on? Ha! You don't want to know!*

~Sally D., *Lymphatic Lifestyle Solutions* Participant

The two most commonly advocated "diets" are "calories in vs. calories out," or CICO, and the Low Fat Diet. The fallacious reasoning behind each of these suggested diets is simple. In CICO, the amount of calories is arbitrarily restricted and in the Low Fat Diet, the amount of fat is arbitrarily restricted.

A recent report from the US Center for Disease Control found that almost one half of US adults are actively trying to lose weight and two thirds of them will attempt to accomplish this by exercising more and eating less food.[44] Unfortunately, following the failed theory dubbed CICO has resulted in the terrible and growing epidemic of overweight people and the increasing number of individuals with obesity and its ancillary maladies. This unfortunate massive nutrition experiment was foisted on the American people with the first issuance of the Dietary Guidelines for Americans in 1977. The result was an explosion in the percentage of Americans with obesity.

This energy balance theory does not differentiate between the metabolic effects of different nutrients. One can lose weight, this useless theory states, even while eating sugar cookies and french fries as long as one doesn't eat more than one expends in physical activity. CICO is not a strategy, it is a description. Surprisingly, this ruse has reigned for far too many decades, even though the science behind it has freighter-sized holes in it.

Removing fat from the diet results in raised carbohydrate or protein intake, both of which trigger larger insulin responses.

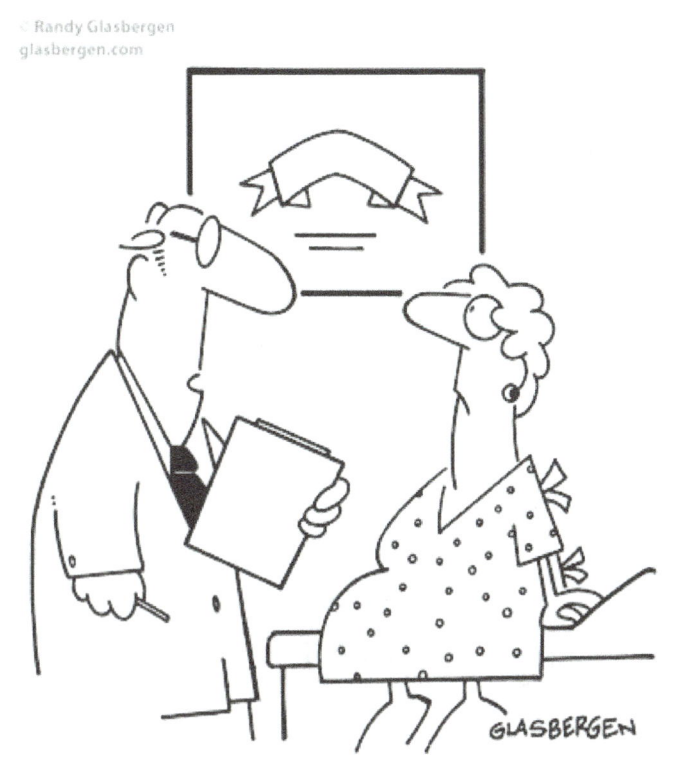

"The high-carb diet I put you on 20 years ago gave you diabetes, high blood pressure and heart disease. Oops."

*Used with permission.*

Since the body can't burn and store fat simultaneously, when insulin is present the body must store fat, the opposite of the desired outcome of a weight loss diet. Increased sequestration of energy by insulin (removal of sugar in the blood to be stored as fat) then leads to hunger, causing the high carbohydrate dieter to eat sooner rather than later in a futile effort to keep their energy level from crashing.

Most of your overweight clients have tried and failed to lower their body weight using caloric restriction. They have not succeeded because calorie restriction is simply a form of medically supervised starvation and as such is unsustainable. Eventually, through no fault of their own, those using this method of dieting will give in to their bodies' desperate hunger for missing

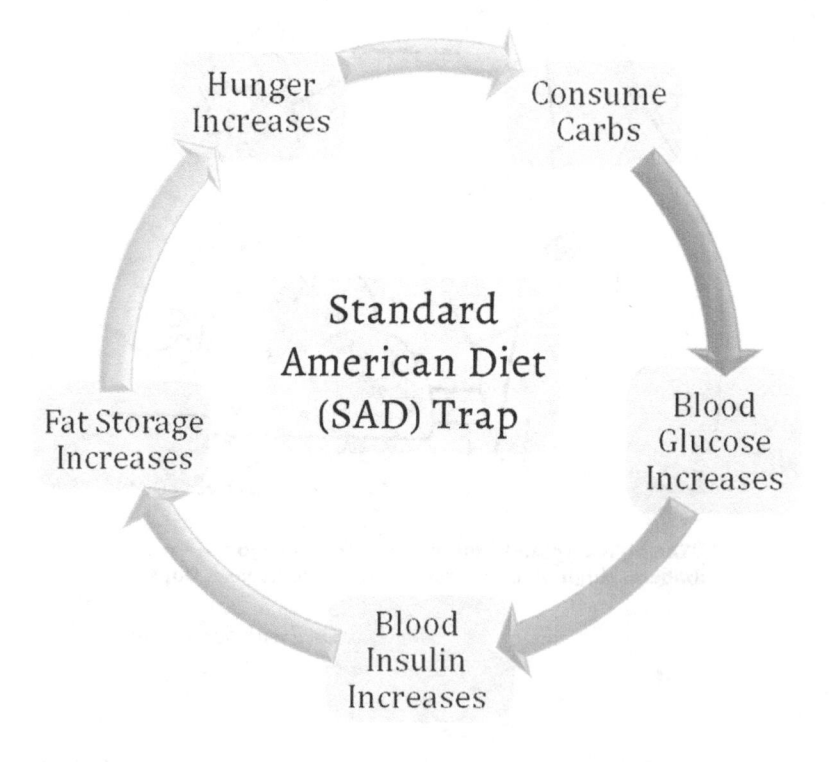

```
        Hunger              Consume
       Increases             Carbs

                  Standard
                American Diet              Blood
 Fat Storage      (SAD) Trap              Glucose
 Increases                                Increases

                    Blood
                   Insulin
                  Increases
```

*Figure 6. The Standard American Diet (SAD) traps people in this vicious carbohydrate cycle. Intake of carbs causes blood sugar to increase and induces the release of insulin. Insulin immediately stops fat burning and encourages fat storage, while triggering hunger because blood sugar has dropped so low. This prompts the intake of more carbs. (Adapted from a presentation by Dr. Sarah Hallberg).*

## It's Like This...

*Gary Taubes uses the analogy of a bar with lots of people inside. Saying that it is crowded because more people came in than went out is not addressing the reasons why more people came in than went out. Maybe the movie next to the bar just let out. Maybe people were enticed to enter because it was happy hour. Establishing the cause is key to developing effective treatment strategies.*

*An analogy Dr. Stephen Phinney uses regarding caloric restriction is this: if you ask someone to hold their breath for any length of time, when the person starts breathing again they will take in as much air as they missed out on during the time they didn't get air. That is a biological imperative. A body needs a certain amount of air just as it needs a certain amount of nutrients. It will struggle to attain those, no matter how miserable the person becomes. At some point, the person will succumb to gasping for air, or with an eating binge in the body's effort to obtain the air or nutrition it has been deprived of.*

nutrients. Most often, this severe deprivation leads to binging on high-carbohydrate foods.

Therapists of all kinds have an ongoing struggle with clients regarding compliance. For many reasons, clients will nod in agreement with a therapist at one appointment, then at that client's next appointment, the therapist finds out that the client has not followed one or more of the protocols of their home program. In lymphedema therapy treatment, this lack of adherence might manifest as the client not keeping compression wraps on or that they are not being diligent with skin care. In conventional weight-management programs or schemes, participants commonly do not follow through because there is no way that eating less and moving more is sustainable in the long term. Exercise, though it has other benefits, makes a person hungrier. For obvious reasons, a person carrying 100 or more extra pounds will find it nigh on impossible to move enough to effect any significant change, and such movement may cause pain, or worse, exacerbate damage to bodily structures.

The failure of CICO has been further demonstrated in several studies using hypocaloric diets.[45-47] Participants using a diet that was calorie-restricted but comprised of an abundance of carbohydrates tended to regain most of their weight. Further, animal studies have repeatedly shown that a predisposition to weight increase is often independent of caloric restriction. This also begs the question of whether obese people must stay on the caloric restriction for the rest of their lives - an impossible endeavor.

Weight loss programs run the gamut from a simple grapefruit diet to complicated diet programs requiring clients to meditate in a yurt in the Arizona desert while sipping exotic elixirs, and everything in between. These various strategies can easily be examined and dismissed since there is a dearth of randomized clinical trials, or even well-designed studies in support of them. A comprehensive review of the literature backing any particular weight loss program is easily undertaken, since there are so few high-quality studies demonstrating efficacy. Nutrition studies in general, and research purporting to prove the success of a particular weight loss program specifically, are commonly riddled with confounders and flawed designs, severely limiting the conclusions that can be drawn.[48] Gary Taubes discusses this in his writings.

> *"The most recent unbiased review of this evidence – from the Cochrane Collaboration, an international organization founded to do such unbiased reviews – has concluded that clinical trials have failed to demonstrate any benefit from eating low-fat diets and so, implicitly, any harm from eating fat-rich foods. The 2015 review describes the evidence as only "suggestive" that avoiding saturated fat specifically may avert a single heart attack and says it's even "less clear" whether this would lengthen anyone's life."*[49]

There is one way of eating that has the backing of many well-designed studies over long time periods with few confounders. In fact, in every randomized, controlled trial with human subjects comparing various diets, the ketogenic diet is superior in all outcome measures including weight, body composition, blood pressure, waistline measure, and blood serum values (such as triglycerides, LDL, HDL, HbA1c). This way of eating will be explored in more detail in the next chapter.

## CASE STUDY: RICHARD

Richard first came into therapy because his legs had swelled up so much that wounds had appeared on his calves. He was 56 years old and weighed 350 lbs. He suffered from severe back and sciatica pain ever since a motorcycle injury 10 years before and this limited his ability to work or exercise. The edema and wounds were easily treated in the lymphedema clinic, but every year or so Richard would return with more swelling and increasing weight. Eventually, he reached 514 lbs. and had been hospitalized multiple times with life-threatening infections. Once, after he suffered respiratory arrest, his wife Maria began searching for oversized coffins. The doctors had told her to expect the worse.

We talked about using a ketogenic diet for weight and lymphedema management for two years before Richard came to me full of resolve and completely ready to give it a try. After 10 weeks on a strict ketogenic diet, Richard's weight reduced from 443 to 408 lbs. More importantly, the large edema volume loss in his legs allowed him to be more mobile and experience less pain.

# Chapter 3

# How Dietary Fat Will Save the Day

## Ketogenic Diet for Health and Weight Loss

*"The low-carb, high-fat diet my therapist taught us about really worked."*

~Danielle J., *Lymphatic Lifestyle Solutions* Participant

*"I have been doing keto for one month and have lost 10 lbs. I have decided to add a little exercise. I actually got down on the floor and was able to get up by myself. Before my legs were so swollen that it hurt to get up and down. I didn't do any measurements but I know some inches have come off. So excited. I love keto."*

~Lipedema & Keto Way of Eating Facebook Group post

Research suggests that the fundamental cause of obesity is not one of physics but of chemistry. Research and clinical knowledge, as early as 1872[50] and up until the national discourse changed in the late 1970s, demonstrated that diets comprised of an excess of carbohydrate and devoid of fat lead to storage of excess adipose tissue, disease and early death.[43,51,52] It is virtually impossible for an otherwise healthy individual to become overweight on a diet comprised solely of proteins and fats, no matter how little one exercises.[53] Carbohydrates in a surprisingly small excess are required for accumulation of fat and weight gain. Necessary nutrients for humans to consume in a healthy diet include essential fatty acids and essential amino acids (the building blocks of protein). There is no such thing as an essential carbohydrate.

> *"I'm one month in today and down 20lbs. But more importantly I feel great, have stopped completely my opiate painkillers, no random stomach aches which I used to get lots of, no headaches or migraine which I also had frequently. My leg pain is much better, I don't feel so stiff and I have a clear head. Why didn't I do this sooner!"*
>
> ~G. B.

> *"I've been looking up the references our therapist gave us and they really explain the ketogenic diet well. Now I understand why it's easy to maintain a healthy weight this way."*
>
> ~Sue C., *Lymphatic Lifestyle Solutions* Participant

A ketogenic diet is a low-carbohydrate, moderate-protein, high-fat way of eating that forces the body to use fat, in the form of ketones and fatty acids, for fuel instead of carbohydrate (glucose). A ketogenic diet promotes ketosis, a healthy metabolic state that doesn't require the presence of insulin, allowing blood sugar to stabilize. Intake of dietary carbohydrate, a non-essential macronutrient, causes the release of insulin which immediately halts the utilization of fat for fuel, and forces all excess carbohydrate into fat storage.

The ketogenic diet used by the Lifestyle Medicine Clinic at Duke University Medical Center in Durham, NC includes recommendations to avoid eating all fruit, to limit vegetable intake to those that are non-starchy, and to eat a liberal amount of healthy fats such as butter, eggs, and meat to satiation.[54] The take-away regarding a well-formulated ketogenic diet is: Don't eat food that raises blood sugar. Dietary fat does not increase blood sugar.

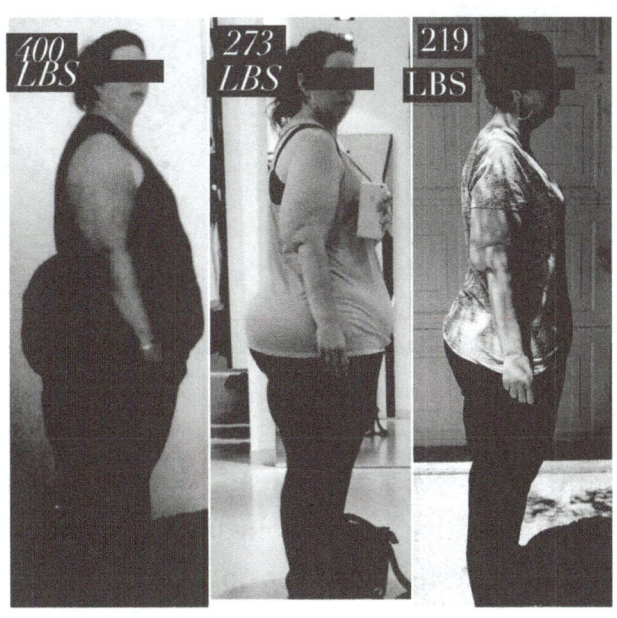

*Figure 7. KD: 181 lbs in less than 2 years "No surgery, no exercise, just [ketogenic] food."*

Despite the tendency of the medical community to falsely malign dietary fat and to encourage intake of unhealthy amounts of carbohydrate, there has been significant recent research that has again established that a well-formulated ketogenic diet is the healthier way of eating and the most successful one for weight loss.[6,8,55] Fortunately, the paradigm is shifting in the scientific community. This is reflected in popular mainstream media outlets like *Time Magazine.*[56] Any concerns regarding the consumption of a high-fat diet were dispelled with *Time's* review of literature absolving fat, including saturated fat, of its ostensible connection to health problems.[56,57]

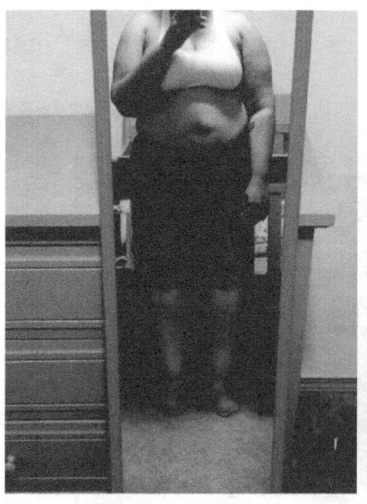

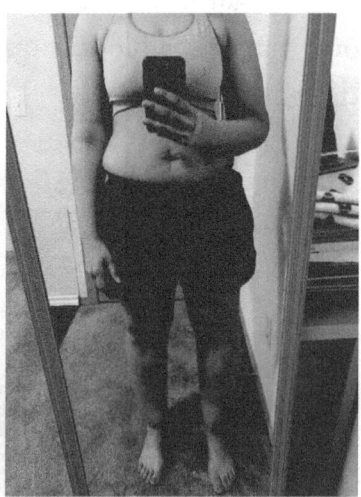

*Figure 8. N.P., 50 lbs. in 5 months*

Over the last 20 years, several studies have demonstrated healthier outcomes with a low-carbohydrate, ketogenic diet even in the presence of obesity-related co-morbidities such as metabolic syndrome,[58] hyperlipidemia,[53,59] cardiovascular disease[60] and type 2 diabetes.[51,61] A review of studies performed from 2002 to 2006 examining the efficacy of a well-formulated low-carbohydrate ketogenic diet demonstrated superiority in all markers of good health including reduction of weight, percent body fat, blood pressure, and BMI as well as blood chemistry improvements such as lowered triglyceride and blood glucose levels, increased HDL, and improved insulin sensitivity[5]. This is accomplished without restricting calories or discouraging dietary fat intake, and without muscle wasting which is commonly observed on low fat, calorically-restricted diets.

The hormonal weight loss theory is called *Low Carb, High Fat* by Dr. Andreas Eenfeldt in the title of his book.[62] Duke

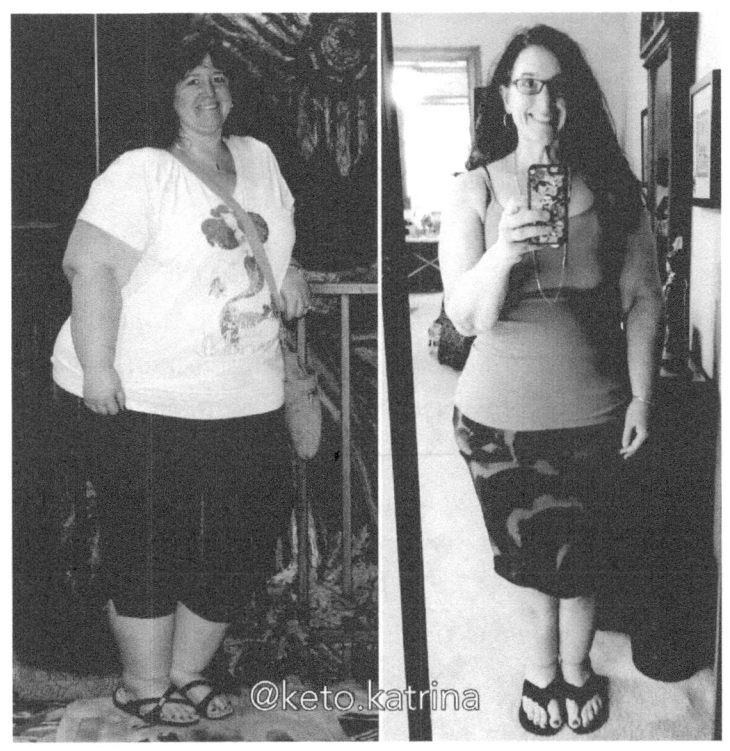

*Figure 9. "Keto for 2.5 years - no cheat day, meal, bite, or lick of the fingers; starting weight: 400; down 199 pounds"*

Lifestyle Medicine Clinic uses the term "No Sugar, No Starch Diet." In Europe and South Africa, it is known as the Banting or Noakes diet. Others have called it a modified Atkins Diet. Drs. Phinney and Volek have coined the phrase "a well-formulated ketogenic diet," which I have decided to use in this book to refer to limiting carbohydrates while at the same time increasing the intake of good fats. Since weight gain is, for the most part, driven by the powerful hormone insulin, the easiest way to decrease insulin and thus its potentially deleterious effects on the body is to limit carbohydrate intake.

The publication *The Dietary Reference Intakes for Energy, Carbohydrate, Fiber, Fat, Fatty Acids, Cholesterol, Protein, and*

## What is Ketosis?

*All human bodies produce ketones from fat metabolism. The rate of ketone production varies depending on diet, time of day, activity level, and other biochemical inputs. Ketones and fat, as well as glucose, can be used as energy substrates. The goal in ketogenic nutrition is to become a "fat burner" in Dr. Eric Westman's lexicon. The level of ketones produced coincides well with the level of fat oxidation (burning). Upon fasting (such as during sleep) ketone production goes up, but not linearly. Several hormones affect ketone production including most predominantly insulin. As insulin increases, ketone production decreases. To raise the level of ketone production, a well-formulated ketogenic diet lowers the amount of carbohydrates which lowers the secretion of insulin.*

*Amino Acids (2005)*, is a standard written resource for the dietetic profession. Even this publication says on page 275:

"*The lower limit of dietary carbohydrate compatible with life apparently is zero, provided that adequate amounts of protein and fat are consumed.*"

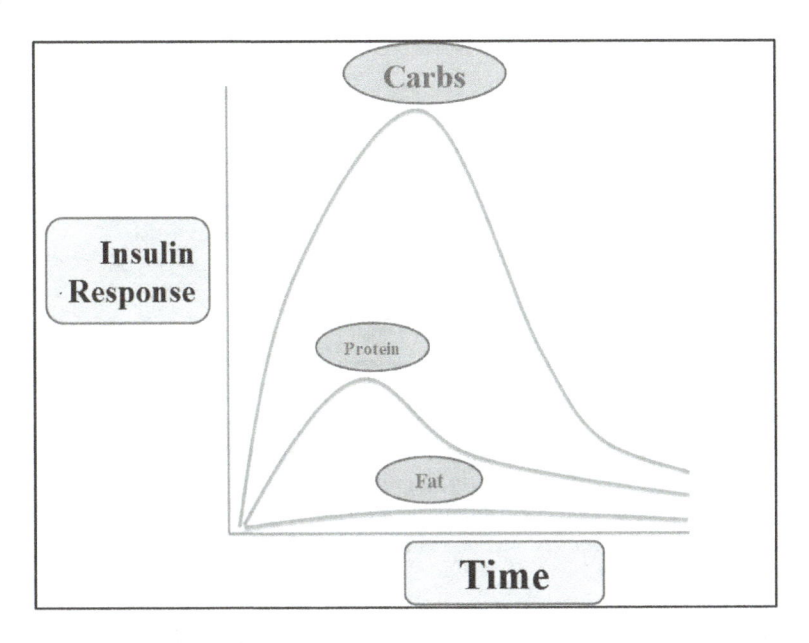

*Figure 10. Insulin response to the three macronutrients. Carbohydrates elicit a very strong insulin response, proteins a moderate response, and fats very little or no insulin response.*

The Association of Nutritionists and Dietitians reversed many years of advice to limit fat consumption when, in May of 2015, they put out a document that states that saturated fat should no longer be a nutrient of concern.[63]

Everybody, no matter their nutrition, creates ketones. Ketogenesis is not controlled by an on-off switch. It is a continuum. Different nutrient intakes create more or fewer ketones. Also, the amount of activity or time between meals affects the amount

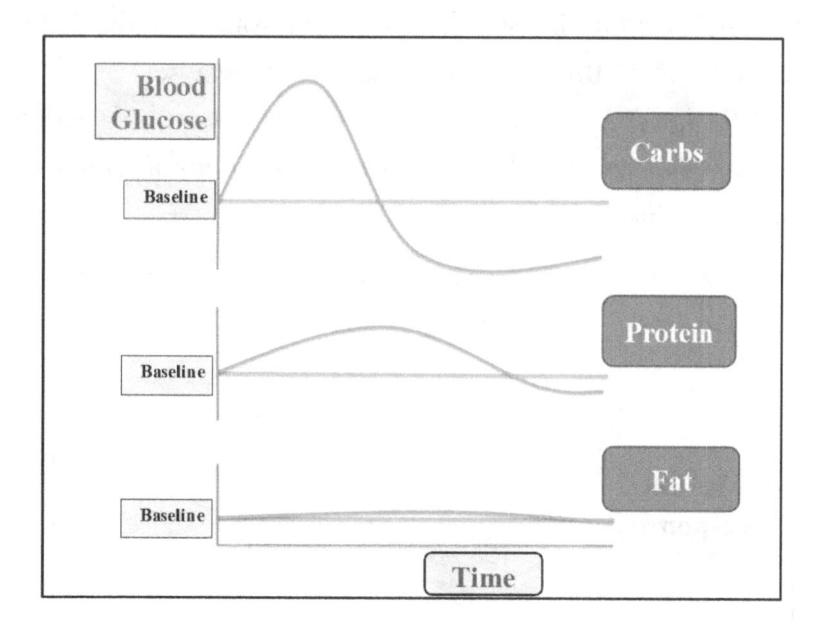

*Figure 11. Differing levels of glucose in the blood in response to intake of the three macronutrients. Blood sugar rises the most with ingestion of carbohydrates. After a strong insulin response, glucose levels drop well below baseline inducing hunger, irritability, and weakness. In contrast, intake of protein results in a modest increase in glucose, while fat does not raise blood glucose levels at all.*

of ketones produced. The aim in a ketogenic way of eating is to elevate the amount of ketones available for use by the body and at the same time increase the body's ability to utilize those ketones and fat for energy needs. This can only happen with a suppressed secretion of insulin.

It is not necessary, when meeting with your client, to go over an elaborate biological explanation behind the hormonal theory of weight loss. Most clients can grasp the simple fact that CICO is a failed paradigm. They've tried it. They know.

Increasingly these days, clients are aware of the hormonal theory of weight loss, but it is likely that they have only read about it in passing or heard it discussed in a derogatory manner. With recent books, studies and internet websites dealing with the issue, the information is becoming more accessible to the public all the time. The USDA still holds to its recommendations which keep people fat and metabolically unhealthy, but the actual studies supporting the hormonal weight loss theory are now available online for anybody to read.

When clients learn that they don't have to limit the amount of food they eat, and that they can choose from a wide variety of delicious foods ad libitum, they become positively jubilant. They may not be happy to have a lymphatic condition, but several clients have told me they are grateful for learning about this way of eating through my interaction with them at my clinic.

Notes such as this one from patient PS are common: *"Just a note to say thank you. After my visit with you, I started the [reduced] carb diet in January. I'm now down 30 lbs. [in May],*

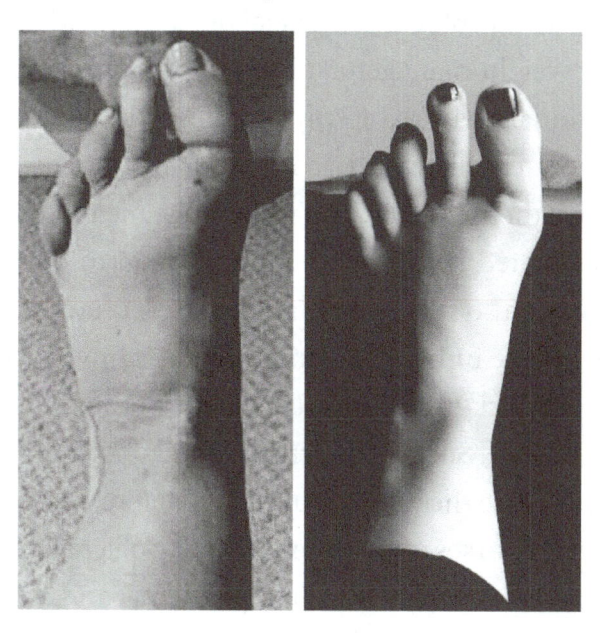

*Figure 12. Fourteen days with a ketogenic diet. Note reduced swelling and improved color.*

with 20 more to go to reach my goal. My legs are better, my knee is better, my mental state is better. Thank you for the push I needed to get a healthy life back."

## Ketogenic Diet for Lymphedema

> "I haven't been able to wear my engagement ring since I was pregnant with my daughter almost 25 years ago. Yesterday, I was able to easily slide on both my wedding band and my engagement ring! Keto has reduced my swelling!!!!"
>
> ~M.S.

A well-formulated ketogenic diet is a powerfully effective means of improving health and enhancing the management of lymphedema. Since I began including a well-formulated ketogenic diet in my treatment protocol, beneficial outcomes with my patients who suffer weight management issues rose remarkably.

Individuals referred to my practice would, in prior years, have been treated solely with a conventional program of complete decongestive therapy. Now, I offer them the means to implement a well-formulated ketogenic diet in addition to the treatment. Some have been so successful that they never have to return for treatment. These individuals, in follow-up conversations, have attributed the lack of need for treatment to their adoption of a ketogenic lifestyle. Such a powerful method of helping clients can seriously decrease the number of clients that return for, in many cases, several courses of treatment. The joy of a patient who had sought treatment primarily for lymphedema, and subsequently started eating a well-formulated ketogenic diet, only to find that he or she didn't need endless treatment, is supremely valuable to me. Hopefully, that scenario would be a confirming experience for any therapist.

The success of a ketogenic diet for managing lymphedema may be attributed to the fact that fat is integral to the health of the lymphatic system. One study showed a correlation between dietary fat ingestion and increased movement of lymphocytes by the lymphatic system.[64] The authors suggest that increased movement of lymphocytes in response to dietary fat metabolism may be a mechanism for keeping the immune system healthy and in a state of readiness. This is one of many reasons why a diet high in healthy dietary fat is advantageous.

Because of its proven effectiveness in the treatment of obesity, a well-formulated low-carbohydrate ketogenic diet has particular implications for the treatment of obesity when lymph stasis is also present. Chakraborty, et al.[35] demonstrated in their research that dietary lipid intake resulted in increased lymph flow, whereas ingestion of a high fructose diet resulted in decreased frequency of lymph contraction along with lower vessel tone. Wong and colleagues[65] propose that dietary fat is essential to the functioning of the lymphatic system and may prove to be useful in the management of lymphedema. *"Our study shows that the usage of fat by lymphatics is programmed in their development, and required for their growth and function. We have demonstrated by enhancing or preventing the usage of fat (or fat byproducts), we can control the growth of lymphatics,"* comments Dr. Brian Wong.

In one study to determine how best to treat chyle leaks, the researchers suggest that by using a diet that restricts short and long chain fatty acids, the burden on impaired intestinal lymphatics will be reduced.[66] A diet high in medium chain triglycerides (MCTs), they surmise, would supply essential fatty acids without contributing to chyle leaks because MCTs, unlike all other fats, bypass the intestinal lymphatics and are transported directly to the liver via the portal vein. Unfortunately, most likely due to the requirement of fat for healthy functioning of the lymphatics, if other fats are in short supply, it seems that the lymphatic system will simply co-opt MCTs. Jensen and colleagues[67] found an increased concentration of MCTs in the thoracic duct (a major lymphatic vessel in the trunk) when intake of short and long chain dietary fat was restricted.

## Keto-Lymphedema Study 2017

Two recent animal studies showed that the excessive adipose tissue in obesity, not a diet high in fat, impaired lymphatic functioning.[68,69] Although obesity and lower leg edema commonly coexist, there had been no studies using human subjects specifically examining the use of a well-formulated ketogenic diet for individuals who are obese and have the co-morbidity of lymphedema until I performed a pilot study in 2015. The results of this study were published in 2017.[70]

We sought to understand if a lifestyle modification program (*Lymphatic Lifestyle Solutions*) designed specifically for people with lymphedema and obesity would lead to healthy outcomes, such as reduced weight and better managed lymphedema. The intervention, held over a period of three months, utilized both group and individual sessions. Data was collected again 30 days post-intervention to do a short term test of sustainability. Results were statistically significant for all outcome measures except for body composition (percent body fat), and offered preliminary evidence that a ketogenic diet may be a valuable intervention for this population. This conclusion was supported by the fact that the participants who adhered to the diet plan (KD group) outperformed those who did not use the diet (NKD group) in every outcome measure including weight, BMI, waistline measure, limb volume, quality of life, and performance/satisfaction with tasks deemed important by the participants.

As a group, the study participants were able to reduce an average of 4.8% of baseline weight, while the subgroup that adhered to a ketogenic diet lost even more (8%). Several authors[71,72] have shown that a modest weight loss of 5-10% of starting weight has a significant impact on health. Probable evidence of improved health for the KD group was demonstrated by associated statistically significant improvements in other outcome measures including weight-related symptoms and limb volume.

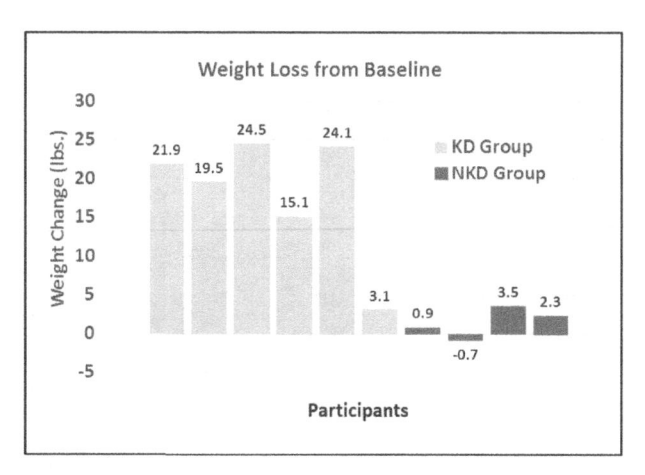

*Figure 13. Individual results for weight loss comparing the two self-reported diet groups: those who used a ketogenic diet (KD) and those who did not (NKD).*

Of note, there was a significant positive correlation between decrease in percent body fat and limb volume reduction for the entire group, as well as statistically significant percent body fat

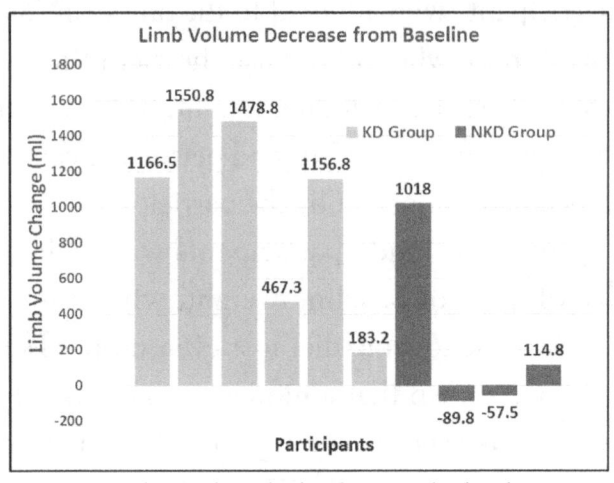

*Figure 14. Individual results for change in limb volume comparing the two self-reported diet groups: those who used a ketogenic diet (KD) and those who did not (NKD).*

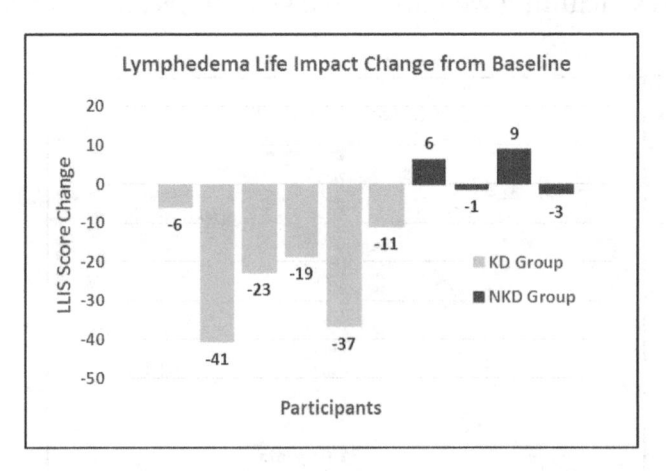

*Figure 15. Individual results for change in impact of lymphedema on life comparing the two self-reported diet groups: those who used a ketogenic diet (KD) and those who did not (NKD). All 6 participants in the KD group reports decreased impact of lymphedema on life, while 2 participants in the NKD group complained of increased impact of lymphedema and the other 2 showed a very limited decrease.*

decrease in the KD group alone, suggesting that, at least in the KD group, fat reduction, and not just edema decrease, had a significant impact on total limb volume. This is similar to a result reported in a study by Ridner and colleagues[73] that showed as little as a seven pound weight loss resulted in adipose tissue reduction in the lymphedematous limb.

Data showed that the *Lymphatic Lifestyle Solutions* Modification Program used in this study was realistic and practical, resulting in a high retention rate (83.33%) and good program attendance. Data from questionnaires completed after each group session showed a largely favorable perception of the program and this was also evident in optional and anonymous evaluations of the full program. Participants revealed they enjoyed learning

## Lymphatic Lifestyle Solutions Program Schedule

Session 1: Orientation/Introduction to Lifestyle Change
Session 2: Eating for Health and Weight Loss
Session 3: Eating Routines/Forming New Habits
Session 4: Barriers to Change and Coping Strategies
Session 5: Prevention/Management of Chronic Medical Conditions
Session 6: Eating Out and Social Eating
Session 7: Field Trip – Meet at Restaurant
Session 8: Physical Activity & Exercise
Session 9: Stress Management
Session 10: The Importance of Sleep
Session 11: Life Balance & Time Management
Session 12: Wrap-up and Review: Planning for Sustained Change

*Figure 16. Lymphatic Lifestyle Solutions session topics. The first seven sessions focused primarily on supporting dietary change.*

about a new way of eating and learning strategies for making and sustaining lifestyle change.

There were several limitations to this study. Because it was designed as a pilot study, there was no control group and a small sample size was used. As is a common occurrence with weight loss studies, there was limited participation by men.[74] Posttest measures were taken only 30 days post-intervention, preventing an examination of long-term effects and sustainability. There can be a potential conflict with the treating therapist also collecting data on outcome measures. Finally, there may have been a participant bias by recruiting my previous clients. There may have been a tendency for participants, who were so familiar with me, to change behaviors or alter responses on self-report measures in an effort to meet my expectations.

## Ketogenic Diet for Lipedema

*Lipedema May Not Be What the Doctors and Researchers Think It Is. Cause or Effect?*

As described in Chapter 1, lipedema is a chronic and progressive fat disorder that affects primarily women and is characterized by excessive fat deposition from the waist to ankles with feet spared, easy bruising, pain and orthostatic edema. Unfortunately, these women are left with the notion that no matter how much they diet, exercise, or undergo complete decongestive therapy treatments, the best they can hope for is to slow or stop the progression of the disease, but they can never be free of it. This misconception is largely due to the inability of researchers and medical professionals to consider that lipedema may be a metabolic disorder, similar to cancer,[75] diabetes[76] and obesity.[53]

I believe that women afflicted with lipedema may actually have an inherited metabolic disorder that can lead to carbohydrate intolerance that contributes to triggering the onset of lipedema during times of hormonal change. If this theory is accurate, then treatment with a well-formulated ketogenic diet would be highly successful.

Pain and inflammation have long been the salient features of lipedema. Several studies have pointed to the excellent anti-inflammatory properties of a ketogenic diet[77,78] due to inhibition of oxidative stress, which may be one of the reasons a well-formulated ketogenic diet benefits a number of conditions. Interrupting the inflammation in the lymphedema-obesity spiral can be why a well-formulated ketogenic diet helps to break that cycle.

A full clinical trial is yet to be undertaken, but anecdotal reports have been highly encouraging. A Facebook group for

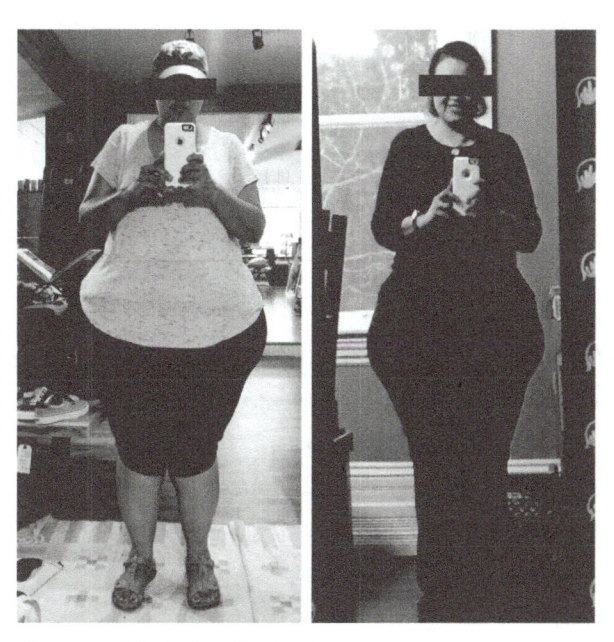

*Figure 17. S.L. lost 49 lbs. in 6 mos.*

women with lipedema (self-diagnosed or otherwise), interested in trying a ketogenic way of eating, was started by Catherine Seo of the Lipedema Project and Katrina Harris of Ketovangelist in September 2016. By December 2016, the group had over two thousand members and two years later the numbers have grown to 7,200. Lipedema & Keto WOE Facebook group provides support from peers and experts, online classes, lifestyle coaching and more. The stories of transformation are inspiring. Here are quotes from some of the women in the group:

> "Started keto on the first of this year. The second picture is after only eleven days!! All the bloating is gone.. If you know how many diets I've done in my life.. this is really amazing!"

> "Doing my laundry and just folded all of my jeans. These are size ten skinny jeans! (stretchy in the leg. But still!!!!). When I started keto, size sixteen was tight and I was wearing leggings, yoga pants or, if I could find a pair of jeans, they were more of a leggings style with almost no structure to them. I'm 5'9" and down to 191 pounds from 251 pounds in the summer and only sixteen pounds to my major goal weight. Keto is the best thing I've ever done for my health and I've even had weight loss surgery."

> "I keep marveling over this WOE [Way of Eating], I am down nine pounds in twelve days with absolutely no exercise other than getting up and making it into work! I keep feeling like I need to balance out my eating more but this is working and it is easy."

*"I have lost seventeen pounds in about six weeks. The pain in my legs and specifically my knees has reduced dramatically, probably 75%. I've adjusted to this way of eating pretty easily, especially since I started feeling and looking so much better."*

*"I've lost 29 pounds. in six weeks. What makes this easy for me now is because I feel amazing. I've not had this much energy in decades. I no longer have any sugar cravings whatsoever. This is finally something I CAN do the rest of my life and enjoy it. I don't feel deprived for the first time in my life."*

*"I'm sitting in economy class seating...wearing Levi's jeans that I bought and never wore (purchased years ago!).. KETO WOE is the only way. I did not fit in economy on American Airlines two years ago—had to switch seats..down 21 pounds [in 8 ½ weeks]. I am sooo happy, I could cry."*

## *A Well-Formulated Ketogenic Diet Takeaway*

*Insulin is the body's fat storage hormone. Replacing dietary carbohydrates with fat reduces the secretion of insulin and allows the body to run on more efficient, anti-inflammatory fuel sources - fat and ketones. Fats are more satiating than carbohydrates. Eating more fat leads to longer spans between meals, allowing insulin levels to remain low for long periods, allowing stored body fat to be used in the absence of insulin. There is no such thing as an essential carbohydrate.*

## CASE STUDY: LILY

*When Lily first came to my clinic, she was in considerable knee pain, obese, and despondent about her weight. She had to guess what her weight was because she had not wanted to step on a scale in more than a decade. At 62 years old, she had spent most of her life fighting her weight and had finally given up. A knee replacement would relieve her of chronic pain, but she had to lose 100 lbs. to be considered for surgery.*

*She had mild swelling in her lower legs, so she felt that at least she could do something about that. She was fitted with Velcro compression garments and we discussed the benefits of a ketogenic diet. The foods on the diet were pleasing to her and her German husband, so she decided to give it a go and a follow-up visit was scheduled for 2 months later. This visit found her with a significant decrease in knee pain and swelling in her legs. She knew her weight to be 342 lbs by a recent visit to her doctor, but did not know how much she had lost so far. Nine months later, her weight was reduced to 273 lbs. And her surgeon agreed to perform a knee replacement. No swelling was present except to her affected knee.*

*For the first time, Lily felt some control of her health and looked forward to a better quality of life with her husband.*

Chapter 4

# A Ketogenic Way of Eating Impacts More Than Just Weight

New reports of the benefits of a ketogenic way of eating come out almost daily. Many conditions which respond well to eating low-carb high-fat also have a swelling component. These include: polycystic ovary syndrome, cardiac and vascular conditions, multiple sclerosis, hypothyroidism and Parkinson's disease. People with lymphatic disorders frequently have additional conditions such as hypertension, Type 2 diabetes, depression and cancer. These maladies, too, have been shown to be favorably impacted by a ketogenic way of eating. The high probability of encountering more than one co-existing condition in your client mandates an examination of how a ketogenic way of eating will affect all comorbidities.

From time to time, two coexisting conditions may appear to require contradictory treatments. What is good for one may be bad for the other. Severe edema in the lower legs and difficulty breathing are two symptoms which regularly accompany congestive heart failure. Recommendations for positioning with legs elevated above the heart to reduce swelling while simultaneously keeping the head raised for easier breathing can make for a very uncomfortable sleeping position. In this chapter, I explore common conditions and surgeries that people with lymphatic disorders and obesity may have and address the concern, "Is a ketogenic way of eating great for weight loss, but not for other conditions?"

## Cancer, Obesity and Lymphedema

*Unholy Trinity*

There is a curious interrelationship between cancer, obesity and lymphedema that can lead to the proliferation of all three conditions. Consider these statements:

- The likelihood of developing lymphedema increases with the presence of obesity.
- Obesity can make existing lymphedema harder to manage.
- Chronic lymphedema can lead to a buildup of fat in the swollen area.
- There is an increased risk of some cancers in the presence of obesity.
- Cancer metastasis is accomplished by traveling to another location by utilizing the lymphatic system.

- A tumor can block lymphatic drainage, triggering lymphedema, sometimes providing the initial warning sign of cancer.

Given the interplay between them, is a ketogenic way of eating appropriate for all three ailments? It turns out that restricting carbohydrates and eating plenty of healthy fat (particularly saturated fat) is important for the management and prevention of each. Travis Christofferson explains, in his 2014 book *Tripping Over the Truth*,[79] what has been known as the Warburg Effect.

Otto Warburg, a Nobel Laureate and researcher from early in the twentieth century observed that cancer cells, for the most part, lack the ability to sustain themselves unless they use glucose as an energy substrate. Most other cells in the body can switch from burning glucose to burning fat or ketone bodies for sustenance. Most types of cancer cells, if deprived of glucose, will die. Several medical practitioners around the world are exploring ways of using this trait of cancer cells to invent medications or protocols to stop the growth of cancers. One method that holds promise, which is being explored by Boston College biology professor and researcher Dr. Thomas Seyfried, is the use of a ketogenic diet. Other researchers are working on developing medications that might sequester glucose away from cancer cells.

In light of the Warburg Effect, recommendations from the USDA give exactly the wrong ratios of macronutrients for battling cancer. A diet consisting of 50% or more carbohydrates as suggested by many as a healthy diet, will favor cancer cell growth. Cancer cells are gluttonous, stealing blood glucose from other cells to feed their own rapid proliferation. This can be attested to by the success of Positron Emission Tomography (PET scan) which uses a radiotracer called fluorodeoxyglucose (FDG) to detect cancerous areas in the body. PET scans graphically show concentrations of the glucose-like tracer and are used to pinpoint the cancer location.

Many cancer survivors currently use a ketogenic way of eating to prevent a recurrence of cancer or to help in the fight against a current cancer diagnosis. T. S. wanted to augment her fight against a recurrence of ovarian cancer with a ketogenic diet. She had a rough and slow struggle beating back her cancer several years ago using the standard chemotherapy treatments. She suffered from nausea, hair loss and extreme fatigue. When she combined ketogenic eating with chemotherapy this time around, she found she was able to maintain her energy level and has suffered very little nausea. Most importantly, she is defeating her cancer more quickly. By limiting her carbohydrate intake, she is able to effectively starve her cancer. She is fully committed to this lifestyle. *"I won't ever change back to how I was eating before. The food is delicious and I'm winning my fight against a deadly disease."*

The preponderance of research indicates that obesity represents a significantly increased risk for the development and severity of lymphedema, recurrence of cancer, and poorer treatment outcomes for each.[73,80-85] In a study of 455 women who were breast cancer survivors, 92% of those with lymphedema were also obese.[86] Some suggest that obesity may be a factor because of surgical complications due to obesity, including poorer and slower healing, increased inflammation, and/or more extensive stress on the lymphatic system with excessive adipose tissue.[87] Overall, it seems that when obesity is a comorbidity, there is a poor prognosis for cancer survival, diminished cancer treatment efficacy, and increased incidence of adverse cancer treatment effects such as fatigue, peripheral neuropathy, and lymphedema.

Fortunately, addressing a patient's obesity with an effective weight management program might not only reduce their risk of cancer-related lymphedema, but may also facilitate its treatment if lymphedema does occur. Several studies have shown a significant correlation between weight loss and reduction in swelling.[70,88,89] A ketogenic diet has been shown to be the most effective diet for weight loss in every randomized controlled trial on human subjects. Additionally, when eating a well-formulated ketogenic diet, weight is lost by decreasing fat mass not lean body mass. Muscle wasting (*cachexia*) is a frequent sequelae to low-calorie low-fat dieting and can be particularly dangerous for people fighting cancer.

## Bariatric Surgery

Weight-loss surgery has seen a stunning rise in popularity in the United States over the last two decades. In 1998, approximately 13,000 bariatric surgeries were performed in the US.[90] By 2015, this number had climbed to 196,000.[91] The large amount of weight that can be lost in a short amount of time, as well as other possible health benefits, are responsible for this stampede toward the operating table. Reports of losing over 100 lbs. in less than a year and the possible resolution of chronic diseases such as diabetes make going under the knife even more appealing.[90] Add to this the very real desperation of people who have unsuccessfully struggled with their weight for most of their life only to still be faced with continued obesity and life-threatening chronic disease. In one study, the most common reasons cited for seeking weight loss surgery were related to health and fear of early death.[92] Most studies show an improvement in quality of life in those who undergo surgery, at least in the short term.[93]

Unfortunately, there can be many lifelong side effects to weight-loss surgeries that might discourage some from choosing this option.[94] The literature reports weight regain, nutritional deficiencies, various complications requiring further surgery, dumping syndrome, hair loss, infection, bowel obstruction, acid reflux, increased incidence of alcohol abuse, and increased risk of death from all causes among the consequences of bariatric surgery.[90,95-99]

The Obesity Medicine Association (OMA), in their 2017 updated Obesity Algorithm document, cite additional serious "acute complications" such as gastrointestinal obstruction and bleeding, pneumonia, blood clots, pulmonary embolism and death. Their list of long term difficulties includes gallstones, hyperparathyroidism, small intestine bacterial overgrowth, kidney stones, anemia, neuropathy, osteoporosis and depression. Yet, given the potential risks of severe obesity, many people will still elect to have weight-loss surgery regardless of this catalog of significant common hazards.

Can a ketogenic diet be used for weight management for those who have already had a weight-loss surgery? In actuality, a ketogenic diet may be particularly suited for someone who has undergone one of these procedures. In order to explain how, we first need to explore the various types of weight-loss surgeries.

There are two main ways that bariatric surgeries work: restriction and malabsorption. *Restriction* means that the amount of food the stomach is able to hold is curtailed. Alternatively, nutrients are prevented from being absorbed or used by the body in surgical techniques that feature *malabsorption*. Some procedures, like the Roux-en-Y gastric bypass (RNY), use both restriction and malabsorption. Some bariatric procedures such as gastric band or balloon can be temporary, and might later be removed, restoring the stomach to normal function. Others, like the RNY, are permanent and non-reversible. Once the stomach or intestines are partially removed, they cannot be retrieved. Patients will spend the rest of their lives trying to duplicate the vital functions these healthy body parts had once performed so effortlessly.

Essentially, resecting healthy tissue is not a solution. There is no other condition besides obesity that requires surgery on normal properly functioning tissue to fix that condition. A nutritional problem cannot be corrected with a surgical fix. But once surgery has taken place, how best can health and quality of life be pursued?

Post-surgery diet recommendations are similar across the board for most weight-loss surgeries, but unfortunately many of the suggestions are not backed up by science or research. Generally, recommendations include eating up to 6 small meals per day, chewing food thoroughly, restricting fat intake, limiting fluid intake with meals, and vitamin/mineral supplementation. Eating high protein is suggested for improving healing from surgery. Because simple carbohydrates are known to cause dumping syndrome, a potentially severe gastrointestinal condition that can occur after surgical weight loss procedures, foods like white bread and anything "obviously full of sugar like candy, ice cream or donuts"[100] should be avoided. Additionally, patients are generally advised to eat mostly so-called "nutrient-dense vegetables."

An eating plan should provide essential nutrients in amounts that promote healing and recovery, health, satiation, and quality of life. All of these needs can be met most effectively with a well-formulated ketogenic eating plan. It can be suitable for most people as soon as solid food is allowed immediately post-surgery and can be crucial in aiding recovery and healing. Some bariatric procedures, such as biliopancreatic diversion with a duodenal switch (BPD-DS) and RNY, result in poor absorption of fat,[101,102] requiring a lower consumption of this macronutrient and medical supervision, but most bariatric procedures do not require a limit on dietary fat. Furthermore, in the initial stages of adopting a ketogenic diet, eating a high amount of fat may not be essential, especially in the case of obesity. "An obese person can get all the fat they need for a ketogenic diet by using their own body fat stores," states Dr. Eric Westman, director of Duke University's Lifestyle Medicine Clinic in Durham, NC.[103]

As discussed earlier, dumping syndrome is most often a reaction to eating simple carbohydrates. According to OMA,[104] dumping syndrome is a "unique complication of RNY" and "occurs in approximately 70-85% of [these] patients." Symptoms may include "facial flushing, lightheadedness, fatigue, reactive hypoglycemia, and postprandial diarrhea." Both types of this complication, early and late dumping, can be completely avoided because carbohydrates are severely restricted on a ketogenic way of eating.

Advice to eat nutrient dense foods after bariatric surgery is fine advice, and easily accomplished with ketogenic nutrition.

The reduced size of the stomach will necessitate getting the most nutrients possible in a smaller space. Food portions in ketogenic meals are much smaller due to the higher density and bioavailability of nutrients found in foods included in this way of eating. Because of the increased nutrient density of fat (9 kcal per gram) compared to protein and carbohydrate (4 kcal per gram each) and the improved ability of the human body to absorb micronutrients from animal products, a much smaller volume of food is required to achieve satiety and proper nutrition with a ketogenic way of eating.

The nutrient density and bioavailability of foods found in a well-formulated ketogenic diet can also aid with micronutrient deficiencies which are commonly experienced after many weight loss procedures. The non-heme iron found in plants is not as readily absorbed by humans as heme iron found in animal products, for example. A great deal more of spinach than red meat would be required to ameliorate iron deficiency anemia, and, likely, such a large quantity that a smaller stomach would never be able to accommodate it.

Another common complaint that is unique to women with lipedema is that, after bariatric surgery, a great deal of weight can be lost, but only from the upper body, accentuating their bodies' disproportion.[105] As seen in the previous chapter, the most effective method - and for women with lipedema, possibly the only method - of losing fat on the lower body is with a well-formulated ketogenic diet. This post by KE on the Lipedema and Keto WOE facebook group[106] illustrates this point:

> "I had gastric bypass in 2005. I started at 460 and got down to 180. I was thin but with thick stumpy legs. I

> *maintained that for 9 years until menopause. Then 4 months later I was at 250, then by 6 months at 300, with full blown stage 2 lipedema and lymphedema. I went on the RAD diet which helped with inflammation but I did not lose an ounce. I started keto 14 weeks ago and I am down 40 lbs. I feel better. I eat small keto meals and am able to do this very easily."*

About one half of all bariatric surgery patients regain up to 40% of their excess weight within the first two years.[107] This is most likely due to continuing to eat the Standard American Diet high in carbohydrates, albeit in much smaller and more frequent meals, after surgery. The same mechanisms that enhanced fat storage and prevented fat burning prior to surgery continue to hold sway after surgery. This very disheartening and common eventual outcome of weight regain can be effectively eliminated by adopting a well-formulated ketogenic diet.

## Liposuction

The most popular cosmetic surgery worldwide is liposuction.[26] Removing excess adipose tissue is used to surgically "fix" obesity and, more recently, some fat disorders like lipedema. Liposuction may not have lasting restrictive or malabsorptive problems, but other downsides to the procedure have been reported.[108] One study demonstrated that the reduction in subcutaneous abdominal fat from liposuction resulted in an *increase* in visceral fat, a risk factor in cardiovascular disease.[109]

In the case of lipedema, liposuction can have the immediate benefit of reducing pain and other symptoms, making it an appealing option for many women with this condition.[110] As with any surgery, though, the risks and benefits must be carefully considered before taking this step. Some adverse outcomes noted in the literature include acute pulmonary edema, infection,[111] lymphatic system damage and development of lymphedema.[112]

Eating a well-formulated ketogenic diet post-liposuction is a great option. This way of eating is known to have anti-inflammatory properties[77] that can help with dermatological conditions.[113] It is likely a well-formulated ketogenic diet will enhance the healing process and decrease the risk of post-surgical infection. Lifestyle and dietary change is required to prevent the re-accumulation of fat in the aftermath of liposuction.[114] Not only would weight regain be prevented, but it is probable that more fat stores would be burned resulting in continued weight loss, if a ketogenic way of eating is adopted post-liposuction.

## Gallstones and Cholecystectomy

The gallbladder is a small pouch that stores bile and then releases it into the small intestine in response to the presence of dietary fat. Bile is necessary for fat digestion and absorption. Long- and short-chain fatty acids are emulsified by the bile to allow for absorption into the intestinal lacteals and transport by the lymphatic system, while medium-chain fatty acids are transported directly to the liver via the portal vein for immediate use.

The most common affliction of the gallbladder is gallstones, which can become quite painful when a stone becomes lodged in the common bile duct. Prevailing medical wisdom has blamed the increased concentration of certain substances associated with obesity, such as cholesterol, as well as diets high in sugar and fat for the formation of painful gallstones.[115] A large body of research also points to adherence to a very low-calorie, low-fat diet and/ or the rapid weight loss associated with bariatric surgeries as the more likely culprits.[116-119] There exists such a high risk of gallstones with rapid weight loss that some have suggested removing the gallbladder (cholecystectomy) at the time of bariatric surgery.[120]

In a meta-analysis of thirteen randomized controlled trials that examined the best methods to prevent gallstones, a diet high in fat was highly recommended.[121] One of these studies showed that 54.5% of participants who followed a low-fat diet developed gallstones, while none of the high-fat diet group did.[117] A suggested mechanism that contributes to diet-induced gallstones is the decreased gallbladder motility experienced in diets low in fat.[117,118] Contents of the gallbladder are more susceptible to forming stones when left to stagnate because of the low demand for bile needed to digest fats.

Although a high-fat diet may prevent gallstone formation, once stones are already present, an alteration to a diet high in fat may precipitate an attack. Increased gallbladder movement may result in a previously asymptomatic stone becoming caught in the common bile duct as bile travels to the intestines. It is also possible that an attack may be avoided because any stones present will be easily flushed out of the gallbladder with the more constant need for bile with a high-fat diet. Medication can be used to dissolve gallstones, but most often a surgical option is chosen as evidenced by the popularity of the surgery. Cholecystectomy is one of the ten most common surgeries performed in the US, with over 700,000 procedures performed laparoscopically every year.[122]

It is still possible to eat a well-formulated ketogenic diet after gallbladder removal. Instead of releasing stored bile in response to the intake of dietary fat, a little bit of bile is released into the intestines continuously. Dr. Andreas Eenfeldt has this to say on his blog about eating ketogenically after cholecystectomy: *"Some people without a gallbladder might have to increase their intake of fat gradually to allow their body time to adapt. Otherwise the body might not have time to digest the fat which could result in loose fatty stools initially. However this rarely seems to be a problem."*

The full blog post can be found on Dr. Eenfeldt's Diet Doctor website here: *https://www.dietdoctor.com/gallstones-and-low-carb#more-1974*.

## Metabolic Syndrome

The most common malady of people consuming a Standard American Diet (SAD) is known as Metabolic Syndrome. Endocrinologist Dr. Gerald Reaven came up with a group of symptoms that make up what he originally termed Syndrome X, after studying insulin resistance and diabetes for many decades.[123] Five characteristics he found to be closely related to insulin resistance (also called glucose intolerance) were:

- Abdominal Obesity
- High Blood Pressure
- High Blood Sugar
- High Serum Triglycerides
- Low HDL

By definition, if a person has any three of these characteristics, they are diagnosed as having Metabolic Syndrome. Metabolic Syndrome is usually considered a marker for prediabetes. More recently another characteristic has been included—High Blood Ferritin Level. Each symptom is considered below.

## Abdominal Obesity

Abdominal obesity, also termed central obesity, is evident when there is excess fat in the trunk starting just below the chest and extending to a protruding belly. This "apple shape" indicates that a high amount of fat is surrounding internal organs and, as in the case of fatty liver disease, those organs are struggling to work under an increased load of fat in and around them. Fatty heart, fatty kidney, fatty spleen and fatty liver are all manifestations of ectopic fat storage. The lymphatic system requires access to properly distributed fat for energy and lymph mobility to run the immune system. In the case of central obesity, fat is not as readily available to the immune protection system.

## High Blood Pressure

High blood pressure is indicated by a reading above about 130 over 85. That in itself can be dangerous, but combined with the other symptoms of Metabolic Syndrome, it means that the cardiovascular system is working much harder than it should. This often leads to heart disease or stroke. Lowering blood pressure is the best way to lower stroke risk. With high blood pressure, arteries become more rigid in the body's effort to protect itself from burst vessels. Sugar makes blood more viscous and, since it takes more force to push viscous fluid around, blood pressure goes up. Carbohydrates are solely made of sugar molecules and contribute most to high blood sugar.

## High Blood Sugar

The criteria for high blood glucose is a fasting plasma glucose greater than 100 milligrams per deciliter. As with the other symptoms of Metabolic Syndrome, high blood glucose by itself can cause problems such as: pronounced hunger, excessive thirst, blurred vision, peripheral neuropathy, poor wound healing and can lead to type 2 diabetes.

## High Serum Triglycerides

Triglycerides are the form fats take when fat is being transported in the bloodstream - three fatty acids adhered to a backbone of glycerol. While high triglycerides in the blood usually is symptomless, hypertriglyceridemia by itself can lead to heart disease and pancreatitis. Counterintuitively, high triglycerides in the blood is caused by eating carbohydrates, not by eating fat. The liver converts excess sugars from carbohydrates into fatty acids, which are then transported throughout the body in the form of triglycerides. Dietary fat is not handled this way. The fat we eat is packaged into chylomicrons which deposit that dietary fat where it is needed, quickly and efficiently without the risk associated with elevated triglycerides.

## Low HDL Cholesterol

LDL, HDL VLDL and IDLs among others are all part of energy distribution in the body. High HDL indicates a healthy mechanism supplying the fats and cholesterol that the body needs for proper functioning. If HDL level is low, cells will lack materials and energy needed for structure and healing. How to keep HDL level up? Eat fat - especially saturated fat. This is easily proven and can be shown within just a few days with simple blood tests.

## High Serum Ferritin Level

The recent addition of high serum ferritin level adds to the mayhem that is metabolic syndrome. Having too much iron alone can cause problems such as cirrhosis of the liver, cardiomyopathy, arthritis and, in men, testicular failure. Oftentimes, high iron levels can be an indication that one or more internal organs is failing. My patients occasionally present with what is called hemosiderin staining, which indicate a high level of iron rich blood pooled, typically, in the lower legs. Again, a simple blood test can show if this condition, a common side effect of excess weight, exists.

In summary, a diagnosis of Metabolic Syndrome is a finding of any three of a group of abnormalities clustered together: Abdominal obesity, high blood pressure, raised blood sugar levels, high triglycerides/low HDL, and high ferritin. Metabolic Syndrome is often called pre-diabetes, but it is more recently being understood as indicating frank type 2 diabetes. There is a continuum between health and full-blown diabetes and if you have three of these symptoms, you likely have diabetes. It all comes down to an inability to metabolize excess carbohydrates properly. And since carbohydrates are never necessary in your diet, there is no need to consume them.

Metabolic Syndrome is associated with a significantly raised risk of cardiovascular disease and diabetes.[124] Doctors have recently come to know what it is and are increasingly willing to order the round of tests needed to get Metabolic Syndrome diagnosed. Fully 33% of the population today will be diagnosed with Metabolic Syndrome.[125] Don't be shy, ask your doctor. I always like to give a positive message, and today's message is that Metabolic Syndrome can be reversed easily and enjoyably with a low-carb, high-fat, moderate-protein way of eating. It's not difficult at all, and it just might save your life.

## Lymphatics/Salt Connection

> "The cure for anything is salt water — sweat, tears, or the sea."
>
> ~Isak Dinesen (Karen Blixen)

Sodium is a vital electrolyte and essential for life. Yet, we have been admonished to limit our salt intake to, as it turns out, dangerously low levels. Sodium has many important roles such as fighting infection, facilitating muscle contraction and nerve cell transmission, regulating blood volume and maintaining the fluid balance in the body. Emergency room admissions, particularly for the elderly, for *hyponatremia* (low sodium in the blood) is more than 31 times more frequent than for *hypernatremia*, or too much sodium in the blood.[126,127] Hyponatremia is often the culprit for another common ER admission: heat stroke or exhaustion during particularly hot weather. A vast amount of salt may be lost by sweating, thus triggering these maladies if salt levels are not replenished.

Most who are prone to edema have been directed to severely curtail salt intake, and may even have noticed increased swelling whenever salty food is eaten. A diet high in carbohydrate causes sodium retention, possibly due to the action of insulin,[128] so typical salty foods like potato chips and pretzels may indeed exacerbate swelling. Because we know that carbohydrate restriction results in increased sodium excretion, a well-formulated ketogenic diet will actually necessitate much greater sodium consumption to compensate for the loss.[129,130]

Drs. John and Judith Casley-Smith, in their premier text about lymphedema and its treatment, are very explicit about "the uselessness of a low salt diet" for lymphedema management.[131] They specifically state that the common advice for people with a lymphatic disorder to adhere to a low salt or salt-free diet is tantamount to prescribing "unnecessary diuretics" and has led to many people suffering needlessly from salt depletion. It is interesting to note that diuretics in and of themselves can lead to salt depletion.[129]

The majority of salt in the body is stored in the subcutaneous lymphatics as the first line of defense against infection.[132] Eating a low salt diet poses another grave danger for people with lymphatic disorders by increasing the risk of infection[129] in a population that is already beset with recurrent, costly, and sometimes life-threatening infections. The increased swelling noted in an infected lymphedematous limb may even be due to water retention secondary to recruitment of sodium used to activate immune functions. One study found that mice on a high salt diet were more equipped to fight major bacterial infections.[133] In a study of ten women with lipedema, elevated sodium levels were seen in subcutaneous tissue.[134] Possibly more sodium was mobilized locally in these women due to the presence of a chronic inflammatory condition.

Recommendations for sodium intake have historically been very low at around 2 grams/day. An analysis from the PURE study,[132] epidemiological research with over 135,000 participants from 18 countries over a period of 7 years, shows that for the vast majority of people, the level of sodium needed daily to be healthy is around 5 grams. Sodium levels above and below 4-5 grams tend to increase risk in people with existing hypertension. However in healthy people, low sodium levels (below 4 grams) show a much greater risk for a cardiac incident than the risk from high sodium levels. This means that most people need more sodium intake, even in the presence of a lymphatic disorder. This translates to an optimal intake of 2.5 teaspoons of salt per day. A well-formulated ketogenic diet with highly nutrient dense foods will supply much of the balance of daily sodium requirement.

As we transition to a ketogenic way of eating, salting food to taste and drinking heated water with bouillon twice a day will help to maintain healthy levels of salt. However, several rare conditions may cause reduced tolerance for salt. For example, hyperaldosteronism, Cushing's disease and Liddle syndrome require medical supervision before increasing salt intake. Drs. Jeff Volek and Stephen Phinney of Virta Health[135] suggest these guidelines for modifying the 5 gram/day recommendation:

1. "People with high blood pressure or fluid retention that persists after keto-adaptation, and particularly if they are taking a diuretic medication, should not increase their sodium intake above 3 grams per day until these symptoms are resolved and the diuretic medication stopped.

2. People routinely taking NSAID medications like ibuprofen (Motrin, Advil) or (Aleve, Naprosyn) are more 'sodium sensitive' because these drugs block salt excretion by the kidneys and raise blood pressure.
3. Heavy physical exercise in the heat will cause increased sodium loss in sweat, which can increase one's daily sodium requirement above the 5 gram level."

## *Low Salt Side Effects*

*The following are some of the milder symptoms of low salt, experienced in the first weeks of transitioning to a ketogenic diet, and therefore, sometimes mistakenly called the "keto flu."*

- *Lassitude and fatigue*
- *Weakness*
- *Headaches*
- *Lightheadedness or dizziness*
- *Anxiety*
- *Nausea*
- *Insomnia*

*If one is experiencing some of the above symptoms, here is a fast fix:*

*Stir 1/2 teaspoon of salt into 8 ounces of water and drink the entire mixture. If symptoms do not resolve or diminish within several minutes, salt depletion can be ruled out.*

# The Malnutrition and Edema Connection

*"Food, food everywhere but no nutrition to eat."*

~(With apologies to Samuel Taylor Coleridge)

Today's therapist draws clientele from a population living in an environment of plenty, having access to any kind of food at any time. One would think that such food availability would result in those clients consuming the most nutritious of diets. This, however, is often not the case. The odds are that your lymphedema clients will display mild to major evidence of maladies related to poor nutrition, making it useful for you to be familiar with diseases of malnutrition. A clinician who understands the connections between nutrient deficiencies and disease will be better prepared to help when they inevitably encounter traits in their clients which may betray unsatisfactory nutrition.

It is commonly thought that nutritional deficiency diseases don't exist in highly developed industrialized countries, and especially in nations that have such high rates of obesity. In the

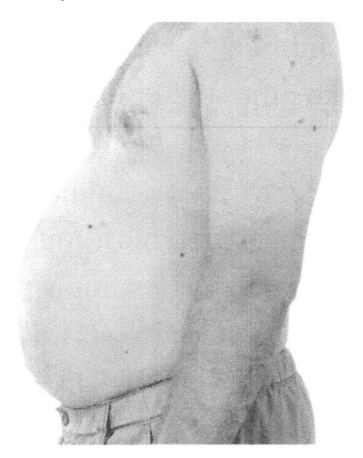

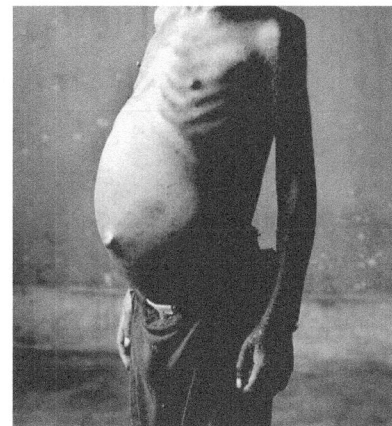

*Figure 18. Are these both images of malnutrition?*

United States, 15.8 million households suffer from food insecurity, hunger and malnutrition,[136] yet almost 40% of adults are obese,[137] sometimes wrongly referred to as a condition of "overnutrition".[138]

It is now understood that one can be simultaneously obese and malnourished. Malnutrition can result from a deficit in the total calories consumed, a deficiency of essential nutrients, or both. Thus, both quantity and quality of food is important. Of importance to this discussion is the distinction that a person may be obese and still be malnourished due to a deficiency of certain nutrients.

Illnesses and treatments common to lymphedema patients may result in malnutrition, such as chemotherapy-induced poor appetite or malabsorption of nutrients after weight-loss surgery. In both of these cases, the patient may have been referred for lymphedema therapy due to lower body edema caused by a protein deficiency.[139] The more severe types of a protein deficit are kwashiorkor and marasmus. Hypoproteinemia (low protein levels in the blood) can be caused by chronic blood loss, but can also be a result of malnutrition. Very low blood serum levels of protein are also seen in a rare condition called *protein-losing enteropathy* in which damage to the intestinal mucosa results in an excessive loss of protein and low blood albumin levels.[140]

Ever since the Dietary Guidelines for Americans first began encouraging a plant-based, low fat diet in 1979, most Americans have endeavored to comply, believing they were eating a healthy diet. The food industry likewise has replaced real foods with what Michael Pollan has termed "food-like substances"[141] in order to market their products as "healthy" and "low fat." These inferior foods are typically loaded with starches and sugars to boost volume and palatability. Data from over 9,000 participants in a 2009-2010 NHANES study found that almost 60% of calories consumed daily came from ultra-processed foods. This accounted for an astounding 90% of all sugar and starch consumed.[142] Unfortunately, a diet high in carbohydrate, as encouraged by the Dietary Guidelines, will so severely displace protein consumption that hypoproteinemia is the inevitable outcome.

*Kwashiorkor* is a condition that is most commonly connected with starvation in developing countries. It is malnutrition of protein intake but with adequate total calories and energy, or carbohydrate, intake. However, it is important to note that anyone can develop kwashiorkor if their diet consists mainly of carbohydrates.[143,144] Kwashiorkor symptoms often include: depression, irritability, tingling in hands and feet, difficulty fighting infection, protruding abdomen, and edema (particularly in the lower body).

*Marasmus* occurs with an inadequate caloric and energy intake. For this reason, a standard low-fat, low-calorie weight-loss diet can result in marasmus if maintained over an extended period of time. A diet high in protein and very low in fat results in *rabbit starvation*. Both marasmus and rabbit starvation can be ameliorated with adequate fat consumption, but often are not associated with peripheral edema.[143]

Lymphedema patients often get repeated bouts of cellulitis and other infections possibly due to difficulty transporting immune components to the infection site in a malformed or damaged lymphatic system. However, another cause of infection may be based more in poor nutrition. Malnutrition exponentially increases the risk of infection and infectious disease and can weaken every part of the immune system.[145] Not only is sufficient salt intake necessary (Chapter 4), but we now know that the lymphatic system needs fat to perform its vital immune functions.[65,146]

Recommendations to eat a plant-based, carbohydrate-heavy diet has led to lower than optimal intake of fat and animal-based foods. Limited intake of fat induces a deficiency of fat soluble micronutrients, such as vitamins A, D, E and K. These vitamins require satisfactory dietary fat to allow for their absorption. Too little of these micronutrients impact immune function (Vitamin A and D), muscle strength (D and E), bone integrity (Vitamin D and K) and heart health (Vitamin K). Additionally, animal-based foods contain many micronutrients which are more bioavailable for use by human bodies and usually in larger quantities as well. The continued insistence on a plant-based diet has led to less than optimal absorption of essential micronutrients for many people.

Another issue to consider is that plants have what are called anti-nutrients, also called phytonutrients, which can block the metabolism of certain essential nutrients, causing deficiencies. Salicylates, phytic acid (or phytates), lignans, saponins, phytoestrogens, oxalates and phenolic compounds - found especially in grains, beans, legumes and nuts — can interfere with adequate absorption of vitamins and minerals.[147] Some lectins as well as protease inhibitors found in plants can cause digestive problems.[148]

Nutrient deficiencies may also be medication-related. For example, a client suffering from gastroesophageal reflux disease (GERD) or heartburn, may be taking Zantac, Prilosec or Omeprazole on a daily basis for an extended period of time.

Stomach acid is necessary for the breakdown of foods in the gut to make available the most nutrition possible. These heartburn medications reduce stomach acid, compromising digestion and absorption of what has been eaten. For clients with diabetes, their insulin and oral diabetes medication can cause intestinal edema.[149] Intestinal edema obstructs the absorption of CoQ10, an exceedingly necessary nutrient for heart health.[150] Statin medications are also well-known to disrupt the creation of CoQ10 and commonly have a side effect of leg swelling, possibly due to the drugs' effects on kidney function.[151]

## CASE STUDY: DARREN

*Darren was born with swelling in both of his legs, with his left leg much more severe. At 64 years old, he was investigating treatment for his lymphedema for the first time in his life. Accommodations had been made for the size of his legs with special clothes, but the weight of his legs made his job as a building contractor challenging.*

*One thing we discussed on his first appointment was how his lymphedema was exacerbated by his almost 300 lbs. of weight.*

*Currently without insurance, he elected to wait to have treatment until he received Medicare the following year. In the meantime, Darren was provided with information on the ketogenic diet. Unbeknownst to me, Darren decided to try this way of eating 4 months prior to our next appointment.*

*In this short time, his weight reduced to 255 lbs., but more astounding was the impact on his legs. The volume of his right leg reduced 17.5% and his left 23.4% without any treatment. The only change Darren made was to his diet. He continues to lose and now reports that he is able to crouch or climb ladders with ease and is enjoying wearing Levis for the first time!*

# Chapter 5

# How Keto Can Change Your Practice

## Scope of Practice: Can I Do That?

Nutritional counseling in a ketogenic way of eating can be a particularly powerful tool in a practice devoted to lymphatic disorders, but many lymphedema therapists are concerned that giving dietary advice may be outside of their scope of practice. Dietary coaching is well within the scope of all health professions, and it may even be considered a duty of care to provide healthy lifestyle advice to promote wellness. This means that instructing clients on healthy eating is not only justifiable, but imperative. When seen through the perspective of not only managing an acute episode of illness, but in the context of a person's whole life as well, providing dietary advice becomes essential. Indeed, "nutrition optimization" and "weight management" are seen as crucial components for health promotion.[152] For someone with obesity and a lymphatic disorder, a healthy eating plan is vital information.

The fact remains that many health professionals may believe their training has not provided them with adequate preparation for making detailed dietary recommendations to patients.[153] For this reason, an interdisciplinary approach is strongly supported to address gaps in training or knowledge.[154] Health care professionals treating lymphatic disorders are typically massage therapists, occupational therapists and physical therapists. Many medical doctors, health coaches, athletic trainers, speech and language pathologists, naturopaths, and registered nurses are increasingly being employed in the treatment of lymphatic disorders. However, even with a good foundation in the science of nutrition and interdisciplinary collaboration, it is necessary to understand if dietary counseling is within a particular discipline's scope of practice.

It's disappointing to see that in a survey of occupational therapists in New South Wales, Australia, it was found that a majority of occupational therapy practitioners did not think that weight management intervention is within the occupational therapy (OT) scope of practice, despite a belief that over one half of the clients they serve are obese.[155] Haracz and colleagues[156] found, in their literature review, that the predominant focus of occupational therapy intervention in obesity treatment was "health promotion and prevention, increasing physical activity participation, modifying dietary intake and reducing the impact of obesity," which suggests that even if an OT might be uncomfortable discussing diet with their clients, it is within the scope of practice.

Physical therapy practitioners as well have noted an important role of nutrition for wound healing, injury rehabilitation, preservation of muscle, weight loss, and disease prevention and management. The official position of the American Physical Therapy Association (House of Delegates P06-15-22-17) is that "the role of the physical therapist to screen for and provide information on diet and nutritional issues to patients, clients, and the community is within the scope of physical therapist practice."[157]

Several health professions are accepted as having a foundation in biological sciences that allow them to provide dietary counseling. These include medical doctors, registered nurses and naturopaths. However, dieticians are the only health profession in which the training and intervention is solely devoted to the management of diet based on a person's individual needs. Each country, province or state may or may not have restrictions on who is allowed to use nutrition as a tool in their practice. It is important to know how the provision of nutritional advice is regulated in the state or region in which you practice.

If you practice in the United States, the Center for Nutrition Advocacy (CNA) provides a starting point to discover what the regulations are in each state. The mission of this organization is "to advance the pivotal role of nutrition practitioners in healthcare through public and private policy." CNA believes that nutritional knowledge is too important for general health to allow it to be restricted to a single discipline. Links to state laws and other information regarding the use of nutrition in

## *Circumstances or Contexts for Nutrition Practice*

- **You are Licensed as Nutritionist/Dietitian** - *You are a nutritionist and/or Dietitian whose academic training, professional credential, and professional experience meet the law's specifications to be licensed in your state*
- **Your Healthcare License Includes Nutrition** - *Your profession is licensed in your state and your defined scope of practice includes language outlining the use of specific nutrition tools as part of your practice (e.g. dietary counseling, supplements, herbal therapy).*
- **Your Healthcare License is Exempt from Nutrition Law** - *Your profession is licensed in your state and the nutrition law contains an exemption for "licensed health professionals" in general, or your profession specifically, to freely use nutrition tools, or to use nutrition tools as an adjunct to your primary profession.*
- **You Are Exempt From Licensure** - *Your profession or work in the community is not licensed but you are identified in the state nutrition law as being exempt from requiring a nutrition license to use some or all stated nutrition tools; or*
- **Nutrition Care is not Criminalized** - *The nutrition licensure law does not criminalize people who do not have the license but rather protects the use of the titles Nutritionist and/or Dietician, or there is no licensure law for nutrition in your state.*
- *(Available at http://nutritionadvocacy.org/your-profession)*

clinical practice can be found at the CNA website address in the sidebar box above. As of June 2018, there are 12 states that have no restrictions at all on who may provide nutritional counseling.

Another 17 states allow only registered dietitians to be licensed, but still allow all health professionals to give dietary advice. In six states, it is illegal to provide dietary advice unless licensed or exempt. The remaining 17 states allow only registered dieticians to provide dietary advice.

## The Power of Group Intervention

A behavioral approach is possibly the most essential component to lifestyle change and weight management.[158] A review of the literature regarding lifestyle modification groups for weight management reveals an approach that provides support for the greatest number of people at the lowest cost, with weight-loss outcomes being sustained for the longest time if continued contact is provided.[72,159] Research has shown that lifestyle modification programs that provide multiple modes of support and guidance for healthy behavior change can be the most successful formula. These modes may include classroom-style lecture, group discussions and activities, application of skills learned in real life situations,[160] and social support and community involvement,[161] sometimes combined with pharmacotherapy.[162]

Although more effective than individual sessions alone, the evidence for positive and sustained outcomes after group-based lifestyle intervention concludes is mixed. Both Ash et al.[163] and Wadden et al.[164] reported that weight loss and healthy behaviors were better maintained by volunteers who had participated in a lifestyle group. Riebe et al.[72] demonstrated that participants in group-based intervention were only able to sustain 48% of initial weight loss over the two year period of the study. However, Foster et al.[165] suggest that the contribution of a group behavioral treatment was essential to maintenance of 63% of initial weight loss at two years in their research. Participants who received a commercial group-based intervention were able to sustain 60% of weight lost over two years, while those in the self-help group regained all the initial weight lost by the conclusion of the study performed by Heshka and colleagues.[166]

Although a low-carbohydrate ketogenic diet has been demonstrated to be effective in the treatment of obesity, many factors prevent individuals from changing their behavior and adhering to a life-long weight management program. Individuals may find it difficult to change, even when faced with a potentially fatal health condition.[167] Without substantial support that can be provided by a lifestyle group, sustaining necessary changes may prove to be very difficult, particularly when choosing to engage in eating patterns that are outside of the norm or even against mainstream medical advice.

Studies examining the effectiveness of behavior modification groups that promote lifestyle change have shown the groups to be the best approach for participants wanting to lose weight.[72,162,163] It has also been shown that such groups may facilitate a modest weight loss of 5-10% of starting weight, which will have a significant impact on health.[71,72]

In my own research using a lifestyle modification group to support adoption of a ketogenic diet,[70] a desire for support from others was highlighted in participant responses on the Full Course Evaluation. Five participants commented that they wished for a longer time for each group session, mostly to allow for more sharing, reflection, and support from each other. Three participants responded to another question by again stating the desire for more time to hear the stories of other participants and to share "successes and struggles." Another noted the wish for "more time" and a "wish to know everyone better." One of the powerful aspects of group treatment is that members no longer have to feel isolated, but instead are supported. This may be accomplished by listening to and sharing stories.[160] Several studies have found group treatment for obesity to be more successful than individual sessions alone.[159,163,166] The results of my own study (see Chapter 3) suggest that when the two approaches are combined, outcomes may be even better.

## Addressing Weight Issues with Clients

*"You miss one hundred percent of the shots you don't take."*

~Attributed to Wayne Gretzky

*"I was surprised to hear my lymphedema therapist talk about my weight. No doctors or other therapists have ever mentioned it."*

~Mary S., *Lymphatic Lifestyle Solutions* Participant

While all medical professionals should be aware of the potential for fat bias, proper attention must be given to the impact of excess weight on health. Whether an overweight patient comes to the clinic for lymphedema treatment due to discomfort or for the way their body looks, holistic treatment must include addressing weight. According to Neil Piller, an Australian physician and researcher of lymphatic disorders, at the late stage at which individuals finally seek out professional help, body image considerations, although important, must become secondary to participation in appropriate treatment programs.[167]

Clearly, lymphedema and overweight are intimately related and discussing one without addressing the other is non-productive in the long run. I understand that some doctors and clinicians may have difficulty speaking directly to a client about that client's obesity in an effort to not seem judgmental, or even because of their own challenges with weight management. Many clinicians have also resisted speaking about weight because they lack effective means for helping their patients. Once a practitioner has an effective treatment strategy and can approach their patient with compassion, a willingness to bring up weight issues soon follows.

Once the client has undergone a lymphedema evaluation, discussion of the schedule of treatment can commence. In addition to explaining the treatment protocol, the client must be informed about issues that could exacerbate their condition or reduce the chance of a successful outcome. These common issues include infection risk, skin care and other factors. Just as critical, the practitioner must be direct if there is a determination that the lymphatic disorder is being exacerbated by the client's weight. For instance, a person presenting with lower limb swelling and a large overhanging abdomen must be informed about how the weight of their belly on their groin can impede lymphatic drainage from the legs. It may be somewhat easier for the therapist or doctor to discuss matters of weight in these types of cases of severe obesity. Practitioners may be less inclined to broach the subject of weight with a patient who is only moderately overweight. When the client's weight is not so obviously severe as to mechanically impinge lymphatic drainage, it can be more difficult to broach the topic. I believe it is of prime importance to do so in any case.

How does a therapist address the issue of overweight or obesity with clients? My inclination is to let the client bring up the issue first, perhaps in a discussion of lifelong difficulty with weight management. If this does not occur, however, I find it is best to bring up the issue of obesity while educating the client about risk reduction practices for lymphedema and infection. As part of this conversation, we talk not only about how the lymphedema is acting on their adipose tissue and vice-versa, but the fact that they may have been misled about the healthiest way to eat. It is important for our clients to understand that a biological and chemical interaction has worked against them, and they should not be accused of having a character flaw. It should be reinforced that the client is not lacking will power because of repeated failures to lose weight and sustain weight loss. Once clients see that they are not at fault for causing their plight, they become open to my well-documented guidance as to how to deal with this vicious cycle.

Clients very likely recognize that they are overweight, whether or not they have made the connection between their weight and their lymphatic condition. Opening a dialog with them regarding weight will certainly need to be done with compassion and sensitivity. These clients often harbor a fear that their therapist or doctor will just rehash one or more of the previously failed programs they have tried. At this point, the client needs reassurance that both their lymphatic condition and their weight can be managed with a reasonable and worthwhile amount of extra work on their part. The health care practitioner might then let the client know that this small bit of effort can be hugely rewarding and it may even be enjoyable.

Virtually all clients come into a medical establishment apprehensive about what will ensue in the course of their treatment. The vast majority soon realize that parts of the treatment offered by lymphedema therapists can be rather pleasant. Who wouldn't want to receive regular massage in the form of manual lymph drainage? In my clinic, they also soon realize that the program for weight loss can be equally pleasant. I emphasize to my clients that they did nothing wrong to cause their lymphedema nor their weight gain. It's not their fault. They should not have to be penalized with harsh and dubious treatment techniques nor austere diet protocols. A positive, supportive atmosphere can go a long way in helping clients achieve success, but they have to buy into what the practitioner is offering.

## Individual Weight Management Counseling

> *"Healthy choices are based on correct information."*
> ~JoAnn Rovig, CLT-LANA, Certified Lymphedema Therapist and Nutrition Therapy Practitioner

Obesity is considered a chronic condition and thus requires frequent and, most likely, long term contact with a medical provider.[168] A primary care physician may be in the best position to take a leading role in coordinating care and providing support, but may feel poorly equipped to do so.[169] Quite often an ancillary provider, such as a lymphedema therapist, may be the only and best provider to actively support lifestyle change. A lymphedema therapist who decides to assume this role must be willing to work with a client over an extended period of time, long past the conclusion of a typical course of complete decongestive therapy.

Working within a theoretical framework suited to you and/or your discipline can help guide you in your interactions with your clients. As an occupational therapist, I have found that Occupational Science has provided me with a strong foundation for intervention.[170] The next most important component of individual weight-loss counseling is to actively listen to your client and determine a course of action together.[171] We must recognize that we are equal partners in collaboration. Both the medical provider and the client have valuable knowledge and life experience they bring to the therapeutic relationship. Many medical providers fail to help their patients lose weight because they are limited to offering only the ineffective "eat less, move more" paradigm, and they also insist on imposing their own goals on the patient.

The Transtheoretical Model of Change (TTM) supports the medical provider in obesity management by identifying which stage of change a client is currently in. TTM also helps the provider to select the most effective interventions to support movement to the next stage.[172] Motivational Interviewing (MI) is a client-centered counseling approach which works quite well with TTM.[173] Both TTM and MI have been used extensively in obesity treatment research. Both approaches see the healthcare provider as a guide facilitating wellness instead of falling back on tactics that are dictatorial and authoritarian.[174,175] These are skills best attained through further reading, study and practice. Look for seminars and workshops available in your area or find them online. See the Resource section (Appendix II) for more information.

Any weight loss program needs to be tailored to the individual to ensure that the goals are attainable and meaningful to the client. Consideration must be made to include any client preferences and be as free as possible of any particular client aversions. Look to various lymphedema evaluation tools that examine performance in all aspects of life to explore areas where improvement or progress is desired. One tool that I have often used is the Lymphedema Life Impact Scale (LLIS). The LLIS is an 18-question self-report measure that examines impairments in physical, psychosocial and functional domains.[176] It can be completed rapidly and goals may be formed using the client's responses.

Quantifying the severity of such symptoms as pain, fatigue or depression lends itself to measurable goal formation and, as well, provides multiple measures of success beyond weight. Non-scale victories (NSVs) demonstrate that progress is occurring even when the scale doesn't budge for several weeks. Consider waistline measures, frequency of participation in social events, subjective reports of decreased "brain fog" (*"I was able to navigate my way through the airport to find my connecting flight all on my own!"*), less hunger and decreased cravings as all legitimate methods demonstrating progress to the person who is working hardest to improve their health: your client. Have blood markers such as HbA1c, triglycerides, HDL, or CRP tested. Recommend a Coronary Artery Calcium (CAC) or Carotid Intima-Media Thickness (CIMT) score for further evidence to medical providers on your client's health care team who might remain skeptical and unconvinced that using a well-formulated ketogenic diet is safe and effective.[177]

As with any medical intervention, an individualized plan will allow for shifts and changes in your strategy in response to health status, stress, injury, medications or other situations that may occur during the course of treatment. It is not unusual for clients to experience steady improvement in multiple markers, including weight and, later, experience no change in weight at all for extended periods of time. Even if progress continues to be exemplary in other areas, lack of movement on the scale can be distressing. Unless there has been absolutely no decrease in weight for at least four weeks however, this is not considered a weight loss stall. The lymphedema therapist assisting their client with weight management is encouraged to carefully investigate reasons for a slowing or temporary stall in weight loss long before four weeks has passed. Explore these reasons to see if any of them might be impeding progress:

- Change in medication
- Menopause/perimenopause
- Increased stress/poor sleep
- Hypothyroidism/Famine response
- Carb Creep (unknowingly increasing carb intake)
- Keto snacking when not hungry
- Individual food intolerances (artificial sweeteners, caffeine, dairy etc.)

Individuals presented with correct information will have a better chance of choosing the best path on their way to restored health. Clinicians who withhold information from clients based on preconceived unsupported biases and dogma are doing their clients a disservice. Modern technology has allowed the medical practitioner to gather information at unprecedented levels. This ability is now in the hands of clients, too. Clients can reasonably be expected to follow up on your advice, so it is imperative that you make recommendations based on well-supported evidence.

Above all, you are your clients' biggest supporter and cheerleader. They have decided to embark on what could be a very arduous and challenging journey. There may be times they are so discouraged they want to give up. They will have lapses and will be disappointed in themselves. Be there for them and let them know you have no intention of giving up and that you will stay by their side for as long as it takes. When they realize their goals, their wildest dreams, you will be sure that you have the best job in the world!

# Chapter 6

# Regarding Opposition

## Sez Who?

Whenever an idea is proposed that runs counter to conventional wisdom, the burden of proof rests on those espousing that plan. Though a ketogenic way of eating has been used for the treatment of several maladies for over a hundred years, reservations still exist for some who encounter it for the first time. A few of their concerns can be quickly dispelled with a bit of research.

People question whether an individual can get enough vitamins and minerals on ketogenic nutrition. Potassium and magnesium supplementation is commonly suggested to people on a well-formulated ketogenic diet. The concern has been that when potatoes or bananas or fortified bread are eliminated from the diet, these specific nutrients will be lacking. Analyzing food nutrition is easily done using online food logs such as CRON-O-Meter or Carb Manager. The nutrient densities of thousands of foods are available on several websites including https://www.

nutrition.gov and https://optimisingnutrition.com, an excellent compilation of food nutrition data gathered from many reliable sources. Looking at the relative availability of potassium, for instance, will show that bananas (not ketogenic) have about 358 mg of potassium per 100 grams whereas 100 grams of fatty fish (ketogenic) has 384 mg of potassium.

Another consideration in this regard is that the availability of certain nutrients on a well-formulated ketogenic diet is orders

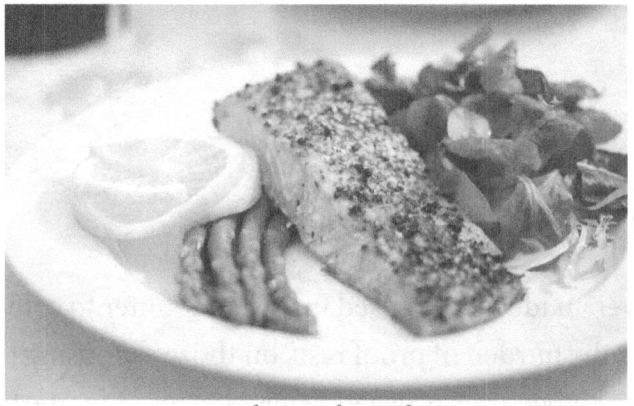

A: low carb meal

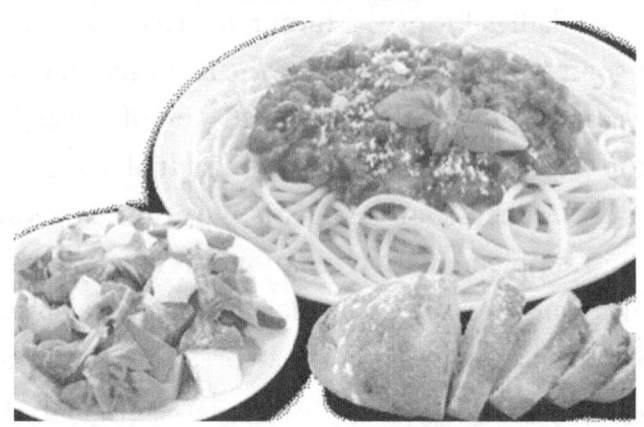

B: high carb meal

*A low carbohydrate ketogenic meal (A) does not look shockingly different from a standard high carbohydrate meal (B).*

of magnitude larger than the availability of those same nutrients found in high carbohydrate foods. For example, spinach contains negligible amounts fat, which renders its content of vitamin A impossible to absorb unless that spinach is eaten with fat and hence ketogenic. It is not difficult to find ketogenic foods that are more nutrient dense, with higher availability of those nutrients, than any high carbohydrate counterpart. Low-carbohydrate high-fat moderate-protein nutrition is in no way lower in nutrition than a high-carbohydrate diet, and in virtually all cases a well-formulated ketogenic diet will be much higher in nutrition, and that nutrition will be much more highly absorbed.

People have expressed to me their worry that ketogenic nutrition might be too expensive. In my counseling of hundreds of clients, that case has not come true. Once an individual becomes keto-adapted, the food necessary to maintain a healthy lifestyle shifts to more whole foods and fewer processed foods. Processed foods come at a premium whether in cost or in health consequences. Overall well-being must be taken into consideration. Additionally, since fat is so filling, smaller portions are needed for satiation. Where a large lean steak may be eaten in one sitting, laden with fat the same size steak may instead last for three meals.

Another concern that does occasionally appear is constipation. This is not unique to a ketogenic diet, but rather is a response to any radical change from any accustomed way of eating. While many think that adding fiber to a diet will alleviate constipation, studies have not shown that fiber will work for that purpose.[178] Dr. Eric Westman of the Duke Lifestyle Medicine Clinic says that adding fiber to relieve constipation is akin to adding cars to clear a traffic jam. Research studies have consistently shown that fat, rather than fiber, is much more effective in alleviating occurrences of constipation and in a more soothing manner.[179,180] Also, people conflate a lessened need to evacuate their bowels with constipation. A well-formulated ketogenic diet without a great amount of fibrous vegetables will result in a reduced need to eliminate. Nothing in a well-formulated ketogenic diet is inherently constipation-inducing. A complaint of constipation should not go ignored, however. Difficult and painful bowel movements are a concern. Make sure the client's electrolytes are balanced and have them pay particular attention to staying hydrated. Many natural laxatives as well as magnesium supplementation can help in this situation.

## Fat Phobia

*"Fat makes us fat just like green vegetables make us green."*

~Anonymous

Because the last 40 years have been dominated by the Diet Heart Hypothesis (fat/cholesterol causes heart disease), concern that "eating all that fat" may be hazardous for heart health causes no little hesitation in adopting a ketogenic diet. In fact, there is no evidence that natural dietary fats, even saturated fats, are unhealthy.[181] Fat phobia can severely restrict food choices. Often fat phobia is extended beyond just fat, and ends up diminishing the consumption of most animal products. This can contribute to severe nutritional deficiencies as animal flesh contains excellent nutrition in highly bioavailable forms, some of which are unavailable in a plant-based diet.

It is telling that certain derogatory language is used in published papers, studies and presentations about the relationship of fat to lymphedema by medical professionals and researchers. Adipose tissue is almost invariably referred to negatively, without regard to whether that adipose tissue is healthy or diseased. Lymph vessels throughout the body are linked closely with adipose tissue, both in anatomical proximity and in function. This is by design. Adipose tissue harbors energy in the form of lipids that the lymph system must have readily available for its immunological response.[28] Only when adipose tissue increases to such a state of overabundance and disorder that its vascularity is impaired can the adipose tissue truly be referred to as detrimental.

Medical personnel must not let their aversion to fat consumption affect their advice to their obese clients. Fat accumulation is chiefly caused by carbohydrates, not lipids (fats and oils) in the diet. The Academy of Nutrition and Dietetics (AND) reversed many years of questionable advice to limit dietary cholesterol consumption when, in May of 2015, they responded to the Scientific Report of the Dietary Guidelines Advisory Committee with a document[63] stating that cholesterol should no longer be a nutrient of concern and that carbohydrates should be limited. This statement follows years of harmful advice to limit fat consumption in exchange for increased carbohydrate intake. That bad advice has been responsible for a majority of the increase in obesity and overweight that has contributed to the rise in weight-related lymphedema. Only by discontinuing those unsound recommendations and urging our clients to obtain most of their caloric energy from fats and oils can their obesity be allayed and their lymphedema be successfully managed.

Ketogenesis commences in earnest when carbohydrate intake is restricted to a small percentage of calories. In order to achieve this, carbs must be replaced with fat. The clinician's challenge is to successfully encourage the client to eat fat as the largest portion of each meal. A goal of 80% of calories eaten as fat will lead to more meaningful outcomes. Contemplating consuming over 75% of energy in the form of fat causes discomfort for many people, even though they have blithely been eating this high a percentage in carbohydrates without any evidence that this is healthy.[181] Since fats have over twice the concentration of energy per unit compared to carbohydrates, the proportions on a dinner plate do not look radically different from a standard Western diet. It is only the idea of such a high level of fat intake that is disconcerting.

There are many psychosocial issues associated with changing to a well-formulated ketogenic diet. First and foremost, food culture in the United States is completely unsupportive of someone who wants to eat fat. Very few choices of good fats are available in typical American markets. For instance, in the ordinary meat section, the butcher's case is almost exclusively red, meaning that all the fat has been trimmed, leaving only very lean cuts of meat. A person must be especially assertive to let their butcher know that they desire the fat. Many people just can't muster this level of assertiveness. It takes a certain degree of resourcefulness to tell someone that they want fat. In one large chain store, I asked if I could get some steak with more fat left on. The butcher informed me that they are instructed to trim the fat to within one quarter inch of the red meat. The trimmed fat is then delivered to rendering companies to be made into cosmetics and other products.

Since the dietary guidelines came into existence in 1980, following no science whatsoever,[181] the nation has been instructed to avoid fat, based on the unfounded idea that fat causes disease. The rest of the developed world has foolishly adopted the United States' official dietary guidelines. Even in the past few years, since the knowledge that fat, and saturated fat specifically, is not harmful and is even beneficial, most of what we read and see and hear still echoes the "fat is harmful" dogma of the past 40 years. It is difficult for people to change their thinking so radically to embrace eating fat in the face of all the false information they have encountered and to which they are still being exposed.

Margaret Mead, a 20th century anthropologist, is credited with saying, "It is easier for a man to change his religion than to change his diet." I have seen how difficult dietary change can be for my patients. Even with regular contact and support along with observing the success achieved by others, only about half of the participants in my groups are able to change. Part of the problem may be the chemical changes that occur in the brain with high levels of carbohydrate intake, particularly grains.[182,183]

Even some clients who do understand the science behind a well-formulated ketogenic diet have told me they are still not willing to give up their bread. Fat phobia has created cognitive dissonance at its most advanced. These clients are saying they'd rather be unhealthy and risk diabetes, heart disease and the inability to manage their lymphedema just to have a bit of bread or ice cream or other carbohydrate of choice. It seems the longer people have eaten high amounts of carbohydrates, the higher probability their brain has become hardwired. This is reflected in the fact that Alzheimer's dementia is now being called type 3 diabetes.[184]

It is also difficult to eat in a manner contrary to what friends and family eat. Obese clients are doubtless surrounded by well-meaning people who don't understand that they must maintain a radically different way of eating for their well-being. This may lead to conflicts in social and family situations. Another psychological issue reinforcing fat phobia in some people is a total reliance on authority figures. If their doctors don't have the latest information regarding ketogenic nutrition, patients will be cautioned to lower their fat consumption and increase their carbohydrates. Many people are incapable of countermanding what they perceive as a directive from an authority figure. Despite her success in losing 35 pounds, decreasing her limb girth, resolving her pain, and increasing her energy and mental clarity, a patient of mine was cautioned by her doctor to stop eating ketogenically because her total cholesterol was elevated. Her physician insisted on treating her blood panel numbers rather than the person, his patient.

Our pervasive food culture, along with existing national dietary guidelines, has likely instilled fat phobia in many of your clients, and their resistance and possibly even hostility to the concept that consuming fat is good for them will be high. My experience is that this opposition is expressed in several ways, including complaints of nausea at the thought of eating "that much fat," or expressing disgust at the sight of fatty foods.

Clients will try to negotiate the replacement of fatty foods with some preferred carbohydrate-loaded food. They may purposely misunderstand directions you give them, or conveniently forget that potatoes are indeed carbohydrates. To counter these ploys, the level of support you will need to give to clients who give ketogenic nutrition a try will range from modest, perhaps once a week, to extensive, up to several times a day. A clinician attempting to incorporate this form of treatment must be willing to have a high level of availability to clients. Fortunately, electronic methods such as email, texting and social media make these tasks easier. The nature of weight management treatment lends itself to these forms of communication and many clinics now use online virtual contact along with various combinations of group support and individual face-to-face meetings. Virta Health has developed a creditable model involving several modes of client support and advocacy.[61] It is impossible to know what approach will prevail with any individual, but overcoming fat phobia is a requisite to progress with ketogenic nutrition.

# Chapter 7

# Ketogenic Nutrition Guide

Dr. Stephen Phinney and Dr. Jeff Volek speak of a "well-formulated ketogenic diet." Here, I'll give you the basics of a well-formulated ketogenic diet. (For a list of acceptable foods, see Appendix II.) The term "diet" is used in the sense of what foods to eat for a healthy lifetime, not in the sense of a short term mechanism for losing weight. Well-formulated ketogenic diets promote health in many ways beyond allowing your body to maintain its optimal weight. Many delicious foods can be incorporated into healthful ketogenic nutrition.

Our first consideration is macronutrients - proteins, fats, and carbohydrates. These are each handled differently, and I'll explain how and why that is.

Most importantly, on a well-formulated ketogenic diet, carbohydrates are limited to less than twenty grams of carbohydrate per day (not per meal). Twenty grams of carbohydrate can easily be eaten in the form of non-starchy vegetables, such as asparagus, cauliflower, broccoli, cabbage or other leafy greens, such as beet greens, bok choy and spinach. Eating fewer than twenty grams of carbs per day is perfectly acceptable, however if there is a concern about getting enough micronutrients - vitamins and minerals - twenty grams allows for a large amount of nutritious vegetables. Dark colored leafy greens have the most micronutrient to carbohydrate ratio and are the best choice for a client's daily ration. If you put kale or parsley or spinach or beet greens into a nutrition calculator, you may be astonished at the volume of these foods required before a twenty gram limit is reached.

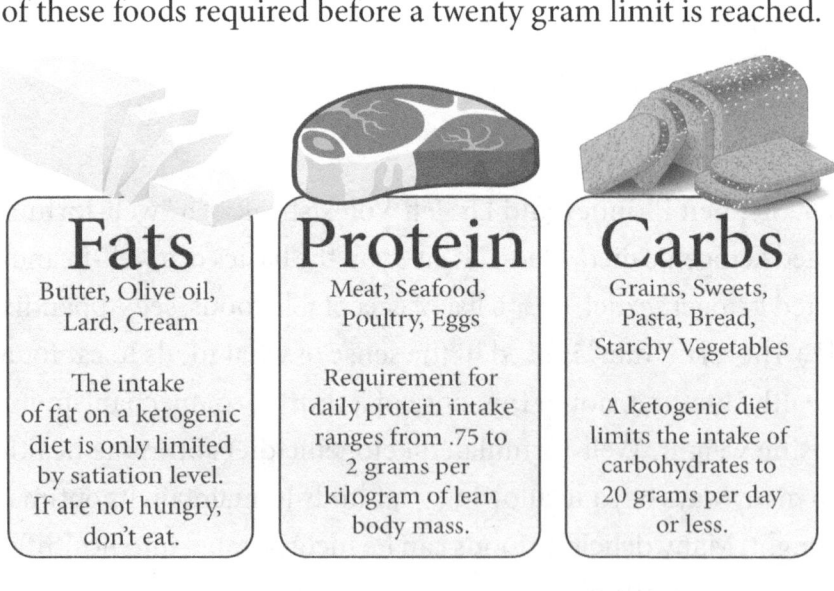

### Fats
Butter, Olive oil, Lard, Cream

The intake of fat on a ketogenic diet is only limited by satiation level. If are not hungry, don't eat.

### Protein
Meat, Seafood, Poultry, Eggs

Requirement for daily protein intake ranges from .75 to 2 grams per kilogram of lean body mass.

### Carbs
Grains, Sweets, Pasta, Bread, Starchy Vegetables

A ketogenic diet limits the intake of carbohydrates to 20 grams per day or less.

Some vegetables that can be problematic to fit into a well-formulated ketogenic diet are olives, cucumbers (pickles) and avocados, which are technically fruits. Fruits are completely restricted during weight loss efforts. Though they are quite healthy, the limits on olives (half a dozen), pickles (one or two) and avocados (one) help your clients avoid the slippery slope of snacking on potential fairly high carbohydrate items. When ideal weight is achieved, fruits, in the form of berries (strawberries, blackberries, blueberries) may be added to the diet infrequently as a special treat.

Next, if we are careful to eat whole foods, such as meat or eggs, the macronutrients in them are generally trusted to be available in the proper amounts, depending on how much we consume. The human body's highest nutritional requirement is healthy fat. Fat comes in the form of saturated fats, monounsaturated fats and polyunsaturated fats. Without getting into a technical discussion of the different types of fats, we know that animal products contain excellent proportions of each of these. Therefore, your client may eat an unlimited amount of meat - that is, ruminants and other foragers such as beef, deer, elk, lamb, and pork. They may include such items as all-meat sausages and hot dogs, pepperoni, sugarless ham and bacon. Poultry and seafood may also be consumed in unlimited amounts. Ocean species, such as sardines, tuna, salmon, shrimp and crabs have excellent associated fats. Lake and stream fish such as trout, bass, or catfish are also chock full of nutrients.

One caveat when consuming animal flesh is that the fat normally surrounding the meat of these animals must be consumed in the same proportion as found in the animal. The healthiest manner of eating is to consume the animal "from nose to tail," or the whole animal including organs, called offal. With few exceptions, such as rodents and other small animals that don't have enough fat to support a healthy human, if we consume the complete animal, we will get the proper nutrients and that nutrition will be in the form of a well-formulated ketogenic diet. In this vein, eggs are an excellent food choice, as they each contain all the elements necessary to create a complete chicken. That is what "nose to tail" is all about, and therefore there is no limit on the amount of eggs a client may consume. Following these rules, protein and fat intakes can be sufficient.

Although meats may be consumed in unlimited amounts, as they have insignificant levels of carbohydrates, on a well-formulated ketogenic diet, protein should be monitored so that excessive amounts are not consumed. Though it is difficult to overeat protein, a recommended limit of protein is 2 grams per kilogram of lean body mass per day. That would be lean meat equaling about the size of the person's fist. Smaller person, smaller fist, larger person, larger fist, ipso facto. And, since the body requires a minimum amount of protein each day to rebuild itself structurally, the minimum protein that should be consumed daily is not less than .75 grams per kilogram of lean body mass per day. Consumption levels must be kept above this for good health.

With carbohydrate limited to 20 grams per day, and protein targeted between .75 to 2 grams per kilogram of lean body mass per day, that leaves us to consider the third macronutrient: fat. How much fat may we eat on a well-formulated ketogenic diet? The rule for fat is that it may be eaten to satiation. Once we have hit our target protein, and had our allowable limit of carbs, if we are still hungry, we may eat more fat. Methods of getting more fat in the diet can include adding olive oil to a salad of leafy greens or putting a dollop of butter on your steak, or cooking eggs in lard. Oils and fats make food much more flavorful and it doesn't take much fat to keep you full and energized once you have been on a ketogenic way of eating.

There is no blanket restriction of dairy on a well-formulated ketogenic diet, but while you are in the weight-loss phase of your ketogenic journey, you can easily consume an excessive amount of such items as cheese or cream. Cheese is recommended to be limited to 4 ounces per day, but that may be any kind of cheese you like, preferably the high fat cheeses that have lower carbohydrate content. Dr. Eric Westman discourages the drinking of your daily calories, either as smoothies or glasses of milk, as it is easy to consume a large amount of unintended energy that way. Cream therefore should be limited to 2 tablespoonfuls per day.

## How Strict Does One Need to Be?

Using a well-formulated ketogenic diet as a treatment for medical conditions is similar to many other medical interventions. Dr. Eric Westman uses this analogy: Say, for instance, you have a headache. If the pain is mild, you might try an over-the-counter analgesic. If that works, fine. But, if your pain is more severe or it's caused by some underlying condition, a higher level of medical intervention would be needed, such as a prescription painkiller. Well-formulated ketogenic diets may be comprised of varying levels of macronutrients. If you're trying to lose just a few pounds and your lymphedema is mild, a higher level of carbohydrate to fat ratio might work fine. If on the other hand, you are morbidly obese, with severe lymphedema, a high level of carbohydrate to fat will not succeed in lowering weight, nor will it allow your body to cope with the lymphedema, just as the over-the-counter medication would not cut the pain from something like a heart attack or a slipped disc. These conditions would warrant a higher level of medical treatment. A more strict level of adherence to consuming high-fat, low-carbohydrate nutrition is necessary to deal with a more severe disorder.

I have been fortunate, in my practice, to have many clients tell me they have reduced their obesity and alleviated their lymphedema using a well-formulated ketogenic diet. This has been a common occurrence. On occasion, however, I'll have a client tell me that they eat low-carb in the morning but eat high-carb in the evening or that they cheat (eat lots of carbs) regularly. Their justifications run the gamut, from, "I don't like to cook" to "I eat out with friends and I order what they're having." As Lady Catherine de Bourgh, in Pride and Prejudice, would say, "I am highly vexed, indeed." Not everyone will acquiesce to this dietary intervention, just as not everyone will be compliant with any one treatment. All you can do is offer steadfast assistance and impart gentle persuasion. You never know - someone might come around after many years, as I have witnessed with a few clients.

# Appendix I

# Ketogenic Ingredients

Lists of so-called ketogenic foods as well as recipes can easily be found on the internet. Technically, there aren't really ketogenic foods. Ketogenic nutrition is defined by what is *not* eaten, and that is carbohydrates. I understand, however, that having some sort of direction, (i.e., a shopping list), will be helpful to many people in their quest to break the cycle of lymphedema and obesity. So, here I've included examples of enjoyable items that can be included into a nourishing and delicious way of eating. Bon Appétit!

When starting out on the course of a well-formulated ketogenic diet, I always recommend that you scrutinize the contents of your cupboards and toss out any foodstuffs that are carbohydrate-based. There is no way to eat corn flakes and stay below 20 grams of carbs per day, so get rid of them. Keeping carbohydrate-laden foods immediately available can erode your resolve to embrace this new healthier lifestyle. Have a trusted item list at hand when shopping, well before you prepare meals.

I've listed items that you can incorporate into healthy, delicious meals. Remember, it is important to keep carbohydrate intake to less than 20 grams per day and to increase fat to satiation. I also have listed several websites with extensive food lists showing the nutrition and macronutrient values of just about any food one might come across. See resources in Appendix II.

On the next page is a list to take to your grocery store. It is organized by where you might find these foods. As a general rule, in the typical American market, you will end up shopping mostly from the perimeter, that is, the dairy section, the produce section, and the meat section. Very few foods amenable to the ketogenic way of eating will be found among the center aisles. The exception might be meats and non-starchy vegetables found with canned or frozen foods. Cheeses and deli meats will be found in the refrigerated section. Here, it must be repeated to choose only those items that you will enjoy eating. There is no need, on a well-formulated ketogenic diet, to eat things you don't like.

## Cooking Tips

*Ketogenic diets are whole, fresh food diets, and cooking can make implementation easier. For instance, you may want to "cook in bulk". Make a cheese and onion quiche on Sunday, and have a slice for breakfast each day for the next week. You can also make roasts and vegetables in advance, and divide the portions into containers for freezing. You will find plenty of recipes on the internet. Just Google "low carb recipes" or "ketogenic recipes" and choose the websites that you like.*

# Ketogenic Shopping List

## Produce

- Leafy greens
- Artichokes
- Asparagus
- Broccoli
- Brussel Sprouts
- Cauliflower
- Celery
- Cucumber
- Eggplant
- Green Beans
- Jicama
- Leeks
- Mushrooms
- Okra
- Onions
- Peppers
- Squash
- Tomatoes
- Zucchini

## Dairy Products

- Full Fat Cheeses
- Heavy Cream
- Sour Cream
- Cream Cheese
- Clotted Cream
- Creme Fraiche
- Turkish or Greek Yogurt

## Meat and Other Proteins

- Bacon
- Beef
- Chicken
- Duck
- Eggs
- Fish
- Lamb
- Liver
- Organ Meats
- Pork
- Shellfish
- Turkey
- Veal
- Venison

## Fats, Oils, Nuts and Seeds

- Avocado Oil
- Butter
- Coconut Oil
- Ghee
- Lard
- Mayonnaise
- Olive Oil
- Almonds
- Brazil Nuts
- Macadamia Nuts
- Pecans
- Pumpkin Seeds
- Sunflower Seeds
- Walnuts

## Beverages

- Water
- Carbonated Unsweetened Flavored Water
- Coffee
- Tea

# Appendix II

# Resources

## Lymphatic Therapy

- Leslyn Keith, OTD, CLT-LANA (*http://leslynkeith.com*)
- Klose Training & Training (*https://klosetraining.com*)
- Lymphatic Education & Research Network (*https://lymphatic-network.org*)
- The Lipidema Project (*https://lipedemaproject.org*)
- Lipedema Simplified (*http://lipedema-simplified.org/keto*)
- National Lymphedema Network (*https://lymphnet.org*)

## Workshops

- Transtheoretical Model of Health Behavior Change:
  - *http://us.thinkt3.com/special-edition-basic-transtheoretical-model-training*
- Motivational Interviewing
  - *http://www.stephenrollnick.com/*
  - *https://motivationalinterviewing.org/about_mint*
  - *https://www.healthpromotionconference.com/*

## Health Websites

- Obesity Medicine Association (*https://obesitymedicine.org*)
- Central Coast Nutrition Conference (*http://www.ccnutritionconference.com*)
- Dr. Peter Attia, Eating Academy (*https://peterattiamd.com/*)
- Dr. William Davis, Wheat Belly (*https://www.wheatbellyblog.com*)
- Dr. Andreas Eenfeldt, Diet Doctor (*https://www.dietdoctor.com*)
- Dr. Malcolm Kendrick, The Great Cholesterol Con (*https://drmalcolmkendrick.org*)
- Dr. David Perlmutter, Grain Brain (*https://www.drperlmutter.com*)
- Dave Feldman, Cholesterol Code (*https://cholesterolcode.com*)
- Ellen Davis, Ketogenic Diet Resource (*https://www.ketogenic-diet-resource.com*)
- Ivor Cummins, The Fat Emperor (*https://thefatemperor.com/blog*)
- Lipedema and Keto: (*https://keto.lipedema-simplified.org/*)
- Low Carb USA (*http://www.lowcarbusa.org*)
- Low Carb Down Under (*http://lowcarbdownunder.com.au*)
- Peter Dobromylskyj, Hyperlipid Blog (*http://high-fat-nutrition.blogspot.com*)
- Public Health Collaboration UK (*https://phcuk.org*)

## Food Log Websites

- Carb Counter (*https://ketologic.com/carbcounter/*)
- Carb Manager (*https://www.carbmanager.com/*)

- Cronometer (*https://cronometer.com/*)
- KetoDiet (*https://ketodietapp.com/*)
- MyFitnessPal (*https://www.myfitnesspal.com/*)
- Total Keto Diet (*https://www.totalketodiet.com/*)

## Low-Carb Health Providers

- Jeffry Gerber (*https://denversdietdoctor.com*)
- Jeff Volek, Steve Phinney & Sarah Hallberg (*https://www.virtahealth.com*)
- Franziska Spritzler (*http://www.lowcarbdietitian.com*)
- Dr. Eric Westman's clinics (*https://healclinics.com*)

## Videos

### On YouTube:

- Dr. Thomas Seyfried, *Cancer as a Metabolic Disease* (*https://www.youtube.com/watch?v=SEE-0U8_NSU*)
- Dr. Jeff Volek, *The Many Facets of Keto-Adaptation* (*https://www.youtube.com/watch?v=n8BY4fyLvZc*)
- Prof. Ken Sikaris, *Cholesterol, When to Worry*
- (*https://www.youtube.com/watch?v=OyzPEii-w0o*)
- *The Widowmaker* Movie (*https://www.youtube.com/watch?v=f1dzECM5ZiA*)
- *Cereal Killers* Movie (*https://www.dietdoctor.com/watch-the-lchf-movie-cereal-killers-for-free*)
- Dr. Ted Naiman, *Insulin Resistance* (*https://www.youtube.com/watch?v=Jd8QFD5Ht18*)
- Dr. Robert Cywes, *Diabetes Understood* (*https://www.lowcarbusa.org/videos/diabetes-understood-series/*)
- Tom Naughton: *Fat Head* (*https://www.fathead-movie.com*)

Videos on the Lymphatic Education & Research Network:

- https://lymphaticnetwork.org/symposium-series/presenters/leslyn-keith
- https://lymphaticnetwork.org/symposium-series/presenters/dr.-eric-westman

## Social Media

- Keto and Fasting for Lymphedema (*https://www.facebook.com/groups/342880423166729/*)
- Lipedema & KETO Way of Eating (*https://www.facebook.com/groups/LipedemaKetoWOE/*)
- Low Carb Support Group By Dr. Eric Westman (*https://www.facebook.com/groups/DukeLowCarbSupportGroup/permalink/1929388043806637/*)

## Books

- Carpender D. *500 Paleo Recipes, Hundreds of Delicious Recipes for Weight Loss and Super Health.* Fair Winds Press (MA); 2012.
- Christofferson T. *Tripping Over the Truth.* Hartford: Chelsea Green Publishing, 2017.
- Cummins I, Gerber J. *Eat Rich, Live Long.* Las Vegas, NV: Victory Belt, 2018. Publishing.
- Davis E. *Fight Cancer with a Ketogenic Diet.* Cheyenne: Gutsy Badger Publishing, 2013.
- Davis E, Runyan K. *The Ketogenic Diet for Type 1 Diabetes.* Cheyenne: Gutsy Badger Publishing, 2014.
- Davis E, Runyan K. *Conquer Type 2 Diabetes with a Ketogenic Diet.* Cheyenne: Gutsy Badger Publishing, 2014.
- Davis W. Wheat Belly: *Lose the Wheat, Lose the Weight, and Find Your Path Back to Health.* Rodale Books, 2014.

- Davis W. *Wheat Belly Cookbook: 150 Recipes to Help You Lose the Wheat, Lose the Weight, and Find Your Path Back to Health.* Rodale Books, 2012.
- Feinman RD. *The World Turned Upside Down.* Brooklyn, New York: NMS Press; 2014.
- Gedgaudas NT. *Primal Body, Primal Mind, Beyond the Paleo Diet for Total Health and a Longer Life.* Healing Arts Press; 2011
- Kraft JR, Fcap JR. *Diabetes Epidemic & You.* Trafford on Demand Pub, 2008.
- Kwasneiwski J. *Homo Optimus.* Warsaw, Poland: WGP Publishing. 2000.
- Masino SA (Ed.) *Ketogenic Diet and Metabolic Therapies: Expanded Roles in Health and Disease.* New York, New York: Oxford University Press. 2016.
- Moore J, Westman EC. *Keto Clarity.* Victory Belt Publishing, 2014.
- Moore J, Westman EC. *Cholesterol Clarity.* Victory Belt Publishing, 2013.
- Perlmutter D, Loberg K. *Grain Brain.* New York, NY: Little, Brown and Co., 2013.
- Simmonds A. *Principia Ketogenica, Compendium of Science Literature on the Benefits of Low Carbohydrate and Ketogenic Diets.* Createspace; 2014.
- Steelman MG, Westman E. *Obesity, Evaluation and Treatment Essentials.* CRC Press; 2016.
- Teicholz N. *The Big Fat Surprise: Why Butter, Meat and Cheese Belong in a Healthy Diet.* New York, New York: Simon & Schuster, 2015.
- Taubes G. *Good Calories, Bad Calories: Fats, Carbs, and the Controversial Science of Diet and Health.* New York: Anchor Books, 2008.
- Taubes G. *Why We Get Fat, and What to Do About It.* New York: Anchor Books, 2011.

- Volek JS, Phinney SD. *The Art and Science of Low Carbohydrate Living: An Expert Guide to Making the Life-Saving Benefits of Carbohydrate Restriction Sustainable and Enjoyable.* Boca Raton: Beyond Obesity, LLC, 2011.
- Volek JS, Phinney SD. *The Art and Science of Low Carbohydrate Performance: A Revolutionary Program to Extend Your Physical and Mental Performance Envelope.* Boca Raton: Beyond Obesity LLC, 2012.
- Westman EC. *A Low Carbohydrate Ketogenic Diet Manual.* CreateSpace, 2013.

# Appendix III

# Lymphatic Lifestyle Solutions Program

*Lymphatic Lifestyle Solutions: A Weight Management Program for Individuals with Lymphedema is available for purchase.*

The *Lymphatic Lifestyle Solutions* weight management program, based on diet and lifestyle, has been found to be the most effective method of retaining an ideal weight and lasting health. Following the program can lead to significant reduction, and in some cases, complete resolution of symptoms. The Low-Carbohydrate High-Fat methods used in my program are evidence-based and scientifically proven.

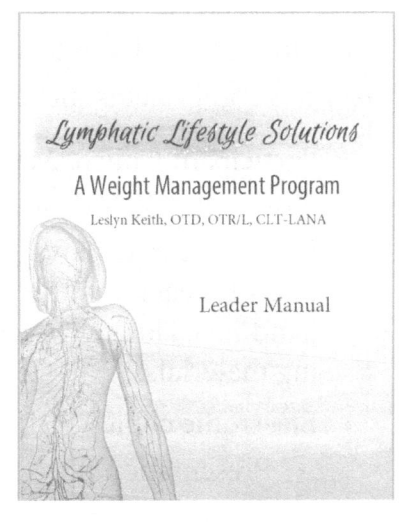

*Lymphatic Lifestyle Solutions* is a fully developed program that is all-inclusive for a clinician to "hit the ground running" with a program designed to offer the greatest results obtainable for their clients with lymphatic and obesity related issues.

To obtain the program supplies with license to implement the *Lymphatic Lifestyle Solutions* program in your clinic, please contact me at leslynkeithot@gmail.com or call: (805) 748-6519 to discuss costs and delivery details.

The package you will receive includes all materials needed to run a professional weight-loss program recommended for up to 25 participants per group, with no limit to how many groups may be offered at a time.

The program incorporates handouts, PowerPoint presentations, suggested testing and evaluation materials, and instructions. The course is divided into 12 modules. The *Lymphatic Lifestyle Solutions* components include:

- Participant Course Manual binder, complete with presentation pages, exercises, handouts and resources
- Leader Course Manual binder, complete with Lesson Plans for each module, all participant worksheets and handouts, along with suggested assessments and marketing materials.
- Electronic copies of the following:
  - Presentation files for 12 modules
  - All components of Participant and Leader Manuals
- A selection of the twelve weekly meeting topics include:
  - Lifestyle Modification
  - Eating for Health and Weight Loss
  - Prevention/Management of Chronic Medical Conditions

- Physical Activity and Exercise
- Stress Management
- Life Balance and Time Management
- Planning for Sustained Change

The *Lymphatic Lifestyle Solutions* program has been developed by Leslyn Keith, OTD, CLT-LANA, an occupational therapist treating patients who have lymphatic disorders, on the central coast of California over the past 20 years. Dr. Keith is a certified lymphedema therapist specializing in obesity-related lymphedema and other chronic weight-related conditions. She is nationally certified by the Lymphology Association of North America (LANA) and is a member of the Obesity Medicine Association. She obtained her doctorate in occupational therapy at the University of Utah.

# References

1. Kohli R, Argento V, Amoateng-Adjepong Y. Obesity-Associated Abdominal Elephantiasis, *Case Reports in Medicine*, vol. 2013, Article ID 626739, 3 pages, 2013.
2. Fife CE, Carter MJ. Lymphedema in the morbidly obese patient: Unique challenges in a unique population. *Ostomy Wound Manage*. 2008; 54(1), 44-56.
3. Ajie WN. My Plate for my family. *J Nutr Educ & Beh*. 2015;47(5): 485.e5.
4. Modell H, Cliff W, Michael J, Mcfarland J, Wenderoth MP, Wright A. A physiologist's view of homeostasis. *Adv Physiol Educ*. 2015;39(4):259-66.
5. Westman EC, Feinman RD, Mavropoulos JC, et al. Low-carbohydrate nutrition and metabolism. *Am J Clin Nutr*. 2007;86(2):276-84.
6. Bazzano LA, Hu T, Reynolds K, et al. Effects of low-carbohydrate and low-fat diets: a randomized trial. *Ann Intern Med*. 2014;161(5):309-18.
7. Feinman RD, Pogozelski WK, Astrup A, et al. Dietary carbohydrate restriction as the first approach in diabetes management: critical review and evidence base. *Nutrition*. 2015;31(1):1-13.
8. Gershuni VM, Yan SL, Medici V. Nutritional ketosis for weight management and reversal of metabolic syndrome. *Curr Nutr Rep*. 2018;7(3):97-106.
9. USDA Dietary Guidelines 2015-2020. Available at *https://academic.oup.com/advances/article/7/3/438/4616725*. Accessed March 4, 2019.
10. Bernas M. The Diagnosis and Treatment of Peripheral Lymphedema: 2016 Consensus Document of the International Society of Lymphology. *Lymphology*. 2016;49:170-184.
11. Szél E, Kemény L, Groma G, Szolnoky G. Pathophysiological dilemmas of lipedema. *Med Hypotheses*. 2014;83(5):599-606.
12. Wold LE, Hines EA, Allen, EV. Lipedema of the legs: A syndrome characterized by fat legs and edema. *Annals of Internal Medicine*. 1951;34(5):1243-50.
13. Varlamov O, Bethea CL, Roberts CT. Sex-specific differences in lipid and glucose metabolism. *Front Endocrinol (Lausanne)*. 2014;5:241.
14. Cignarella A, Bolego C. Mechanisms of estrogen protection in diabetes and metabolic disease. *Horm Mol Biol Clin Investig*. 2010;4(2):575-80.
15. Rockson SG. Lymphatic Medicine: Paradoxically and Unnecessarily Ignored. *Lymphat Res Biol*. 2017;15(4):315-316.

16. Zuther JE. *Lymphedema Management: The Comprehensive Guide for Practitioners.* Thieme Medical Publishers, Inc., 2005. ISBN: 1-58890-284-6.
17. Damstra, RJ. *Diagnostic and Therapeutic Aspects of Lymphedema, Second Edition.* Rabe Medical Publishing Bonn, 2013. ISBN: 9783940654298.
18. Levick JR, Michel CC. Microvascular fluid exchange and the revised Starling principle. *Cardiovasc Res.* 2010;87(2):198-210.
19. Weissleder H, Schuchhardt C. *Lymphedema: Diagnosis and Therapy, Second Edition.* Kagerer Kommunikation 1997. ISBN: 3929493144.
20. Bays H, Dujovne CA. Adiposopathy is a more rational treatment target for metabolic disease than obesity alone. *Curr Atheroscler Rep.* 2006;8(2):144-56.
21. Shimizu Y, Shibata R, Ishii M, et al. Adiponectin-mediated modulation of lymphatic vessel formation and lymphedema. *J Am Heart Assoc.* 2013;2(5):e000438.
22. Esfahani M, Movahedian A, Baranchi M, Goodarzi MT. Adiponectin: an adipokine with protective features against metabolic syndrome. *Iran J Basic Med Sci.* 2015;18(5):430-42.
23. Granzow JW, Soderberg JM, Kaji AH, Dauphine C. Review of current surgical treatments for lymphedema. *Ann Surg Oncol.* 2014;21(4):1195-201.
24. Haczeyni F, Bell-Anderson KS, Farrell GC. Causes and mechanisms of adipocyte enlargement and adipose expansion. *Obes Rev.* 2018;19(3):406-420.
25. Harms M, Seale P. Brown and beige fat: development, function and therapeutic potential. *Nat Med.* 2013;19(10):1252-63.
26. Rosen ED, Spiegelman BM. What we talk about when we talk about fat. *Cell.* 2014;156(1-2):20-44.
27. Cinti S. The adipose organ at a glance. *Dis Model Mech.* 2012 Sep;5(5):588-94.
28. Harvey NL. The link between lymphatic function and adipose biology. *Ann N Y Acad Sci.* 2008;1131:82-8.
29. Harvey NL, Gordon EJ. Deciphering the roles of macrophages in developmental and inflammation stimulated lymphangiogenesis. *Vasc Cell.* 2012;4(1):15.
30. Scallan JP, Hill MA, Davis MJ. Lymphatic vascular integrity is disrupted in type 2 diabetes due to impaired nitric oxide signalling. *Cardiovasc Res.* 2015;107(1):89-97.
31. Földi, E. (personal communication, June 19, 2013).
32. Dixon JB. Lymphatic lipid transport: sewer or subway? *Trends Endocrinol Metab.* 2010;21(8):480-7.
33. Brorson H. From lymph to fat: complete reduction of lymphoedema. *Phlebology.* 2010;25 Suppl 1:52-63.
34. Fusonie DP, Marable SA. Lymphedema of the lower extremity: report of two cases of primary lymphedema illustrating medical and surgical therapy. *Am Surg.* 1967;33(6):494-8.
35. Chakraborty S, Davis MJ, Muthuchamy M. Emerging trends in the pathophysiology of lymphatic contractile function. *Semin Cell Dev Biol.* 2015 Feb;38:55-66. Epub 2015 Jan 21. Review.
36. Wang Y, Oliver G. Current views on the function of the lymphatic vasculature in health and disease. *Genes Dev.* 2010;24(19):2115-26.
37. Rutkowski JM, Davis KE, Scherer PE. Mechanisms of obesity and related pathologies: the macro- and microcirculation of adipose tissue. *FEBS J.* 2009;276(20):5738-46.
38. Aschen S, Zampell JC, Elhadad S, Weitman E, De Brot M, Mehrara BJ. Regulation of

adipogenesis by lymphatic fluid stasis: Part II. Expression of adipose differentiation genes. *Plast Reconstr Surg.* 2012;129(4):838-47.

39. Musso G, Cassader M, Cohney S, et al. Fatty Liver and Chronic Kidney Disease: Novel Mechanistic Insights and Therapeutic Opportunities. *Diabetes Care.* 2016;39(10):1830-45.

40. Cucchi F, Rossmeislova L, Simonsen L, Jensen MR, Bülow J. A vicious circle in chronic lymphoedema pathophysiology? An adipocentric view. *Obes Rev.* 2017;18(10):1159-1169.

41. Woodruff CW. Dietary goals for the United States. *Am Journal of Diseases of Children.* 1979;133(4):371-372.

42. Finkelstein, EA, Strombotne, KL, Popkin, BM. The costs of obesity and implications for policymakers. Choices: *The Magazine of Food, Farm & Resource Issues.* 2010;25(3).

43. Taubes, G. *Why We Get Fat, and What to Do About It.* New York: Anchor Books, 2011. ISBN: 9780307272706.

44. Martin CB, Herrick KA, Sarafrazi N, Ogden CL. Attempts to Lose Weight Among Adults in the United States, 2013-2016. *NCHS Data Brief.* 2018;(313):1-8.

45. Abete I, Parra D, Martinez JA. Energy-restricted diets based on a distinct food selection affecting the glycemic index induce different weight loss and oxidative response. *Clin Nutr.* 2008;27(4):545-51.

46. Jiménez Jaime T, Leiva Balich L, Barrera Acevedo G, et al. Effect of calorie restriction on energy expenditure in overweight and obese adult women. *Nutr Hosp.* 2015;31(6):2428-36.

47. Walsh CO, Ebbeling CB, Swain JF, Markowitz RL, Feldman HA, Ludwig DS. Effects of diet composition on postprandial energy availability during weight loss maintenance. *PLoS ONE.* 2013;8(3):e58172.

48. Weaver CM, Miller JW. Challenges in conducting clinical nutrition research. *Nutr Rev.* 2017;75(7):491-499.

49. Taubes, Gary. "Minimal carbs, lots of fat, incredible dieting results — but not enough science." *The Globe and Mail,* Dec 27, 2017. Canadian Newsstand. Available at *https://www.theglobeandmail.com/opinion/minimal-carbs-lots-of-fat-incredible-results-but-no-science/article37402123/.*

50. Pennington AW. Treatment of obesity with calorically unrestricted diets. *J Clin Nutr.* 1953;1(5):343-8.

51. Boden G, Sargrad K, Homko C, Mozzoli M, Stein TP. Effect of a low-carbohydrate diet on appetite, blood glucose levels, and insulin resistance in obese patients with type 2 diabetes. *Ann Intern Med.* 2005;142(6):403-11.

52. Westman EC, Steelman GM (Eds.) *Obesity: Evaluation and treatment essentials.* New York, New York: Informa Healthcare, 2010.

53. Yancy WS, Olsen MK, Guyton JR, Bakst RP, Westman EC. A low-carbohydrate, ketogenic diet versus a low-fat diet to treat obesity and hyperlipidemia: a randomized, controlled trial. *Ann Intern Med.* 2004;140(10):769-77.

54. Westman EC. *A Low Carbohydrate, Ketogenic Diet Manual: No Sugar, No Starch Diet.* Createspace. 2013. ISBN: 978-1-63002-295-2.

55. Bueno NB, De Melo IS, De Oliveira SL, Da Rocha Ataide T. Very-low-carbohydrate ketogenic diet v. low-fat diet for long-term weight loss: a meta-analysis of randomised controlled trials. *Br J Nutr.* 2013;110(7):1178-87.

56. Walsh, B. Ending the war on fat. Time Magazine. 2014;183(24), 28-35.

57. Siri-Tarino PW, Sun Q, Hu FB, Krauss RM. Meta-analysis of prospective cohort

studies evaluating the association of saturated fat with cardiovascular disease. *Am J Clin Nutr.* 2010;91(3):535-46.

58. Volek JS, Fernandez ML, Feinman RD, Phinney SD. Dietary carbohydrate restriction induces a unique metabolic state positively affecting atherogenic dyslipidemia, fatty acid partitioning, and metabolic syndrome. *Prog Lipid Res.* 2008;47(5):307-18.

59. Dashti HM, Al-Zaid NS, Mathew TC, et al. Long term effects of ketogenic diet in obese subjects with high cholesterol level. *Mol Cell Biochem.* 2006;286(1-2):1-9.

60. Westman EC, Yancy WS, Edman JS, Tomlin KF, Perkins CE. Effect of 6-month adherence to a very low carbohydrate diet program. *Am J Med.* 2002;113(1):30-6.

61. McKenzie AL, Hallberg SJ, Creighton BC, et al. A Novel Intervention Including Individualized Nutritional Recommendations Reduces Hemoglobin A1c Level, Medication Use, and Weight in Type 2 Diabetes. *JMIR Diabetes.* 2017;2(1):e5.

62. Eenfeldt A. *Low Carb, High Fat Food Revolution, Advice and Recipes to Improve Your Health and Reduce Your Weight.* Skyhorse; 2014. ISBN: 9781629145457.

63. Academy of Nutrition and Dietetics (AND) website. Position on DGAC. Available at https://www.eatrightpro.org/news-center/on-the-pulse-of-public-policy/regulatory-comments/dgac-scientific-report. Section V, subtopic B.

64. Miura S, Sekizuka E, Nagata H, et al. Increased lymphocyte transport by lipid absorption in rat mesenteric lymphatics. *Am J Physiol.* 1987;253(5 Pt 1):G596-600.

65. Wong BW, Wang X, Zecchin A, et al. The role of fatty acid β-oxidation in lymphangiogenesis. *Nature.* 2017;542(7639):49-54.

66. McCray S, Parrish CR. Nutritional Management of Chyle Leaks: An Update. *Practical Gastroenterology* 2011;35(4):12-32.

67. Jensen GL, Mascioli EA, Meyer LP, et al. Dietary modification of chyle composition in chylothorax. *Gastroenterology.* 1989;97(3):761-5.

68. García Nores GD, Cuzzone DA, Albano NJ, et al. Obesity but not high-fat diet impairs lymphatic function. *Int J Obes (Lond).* 2016;40(10):1582-1590.

69. Gousopoulos E, Karaman S, Proulx ST, Leu K, Buschle D, Detmar M. High-fat diet in the absence of obesity does not aggravate surgically induced lymphoedema in mice. *Eur Surg Res.* 2017;58(3-4):180-192.

70. Keith L, Rowsemitt C, Richards L. Lifestyle modification group for management of obesity and lymphedema results in significant outcomes. *American Journal of Lifestyle Medicine.* 2017;11.

71. Pi-Sunyer, FX. (1996). A review of long-term studies evaluating the efficacy of weight loss in ameliorating disorders associated with obesity. *Clinical Therapeutics*, 18(6), 1006-1035.

72. Riebe D, Blissmer B, Greene G, et al. Long-term maintenance of exercise and healthy eating behaviors in overweight adults. *Prev Med.* 2005;40(6):769-78.

73. Ridner SH, Dietrich MS, Stewart BR, Armer JM. Body mass index and breast cancer treatment-related lymphedema. *Support Care Cancer.* 2011;19(6):853-7.

74. Arrebola E, Gómez-Candela C, Fernández-Fernández C, Loria V, Muñoz-Pérez E, Bermejo LM. Evaluation of a lifestyle modification program for treatment of overweight and nonmorbid obesity in primary healthcare and its influence on health-related quality of life. *Nutr Clin Pract.* 2011;26(3):316-21.

75. Klement RJ, Kämmerer U. Is there a role for carbohydrate restriction in the treatment and prevention of cancer? *Nutr Metab (Lond).* 2011;8:75.

76. Feinman RD, Pogozelski WK, Astrup A, et al. Dietary carbohydrate restriction as the

first approach in diabetes management: critical review and evidence base. *Nutrition.* 2015;31(1):1-13.

77. Ruskin DN, Kawamura M, Masino SA. Reduced pain and inflammation in juvenile and adult rats fed a ketogenic diet. *PLoS ONE.* 2009;4(12):e8349.
78. Yang JS, Gerber JN, You HJ. (2017). Association between fasting insulin and high-sensitivity C-reactive protein in Korean adults. *BMJ Open Sport & Exercise Medicine,* 2017;3:e000236 .
79. Christofferson, T. *Tripping Over the Truth.* Hartford: Chelsea Green Publishing, 2017.
80. Paskett ED, Dean JA, Oliveri JM, Harrop JP. Cancer-related lymphedema risk factors, diagnosis, treatment, and impact: a review. *J Clin Oncol.* 2012;30(30):3726-33.
81. Helyer LK, Varnic M, Le LW, Leong W, Mccready D. Obesity is a risk factor for developing postoperative lymphedema in breast cancer patients. *Breast J.* 2010;16(1):48-54.
82. Shaitelman SF, Cromwell KD, Rasmussen JC, et al. Recent progress in the treatment and prevention of cancer-related lymphedema. *CA Cancer J Clin.* 2015;65(1):55-81.
83. Widschwendter P, Friedl TW, Schwentner L, et al. The influence of obesity on survival in early, high-risk breast cancer: results from the randomized SUCCESS A trial. *Breast Cancer Res.* 2015;17:129.
84. Yost KJ, Cheville AL, Al-Hilli MM, et al. Lymphedema after surgery for endometrial cancer: prevalence, risk factors, and quality of life. *Obstet Gynecol.* 2014;124(2 Pt 1):307-15.
85. Demark-Wahnefried W, Campbell KL, Hayes SC. Weight management and its role in breast cancer rehabilitation. *Cancer.* 2012;118(8 Suppl):2277-87.
86. Ugur S, Arıcı C, Yaprak M, et al. Risk factors of breast cancer-related lymphedema. *Lymphat Res Biol.* 2013;11(2):72-5.
87. Ahmed RL, Schmitz KH, Prizment AE, Folsom AR. Risk factors for lymphedema in breast cancer survivors, the Iowa Women's Health Study. *Breast Cancer Res Treat.* 2011;130(3):981-91.
88. Shaw C, Mortimer P, Judd PA. A randomized controlled trial of weight reduction as a treatment for breast cancer-related lymphedema. *Cancer.* 2007;110(8):1868-74.
89. Winkels RM, Sturgeon KM, Kallan MJ, et al. The women in steady exercise research (WISER) survivor trial: The innovative transdisciplinary design of a randomized controlled trial of exercise and weight-loss interventions among breast cancer survivors with lymphedema. *Contemp Clin Trials.* 2017;61:63-72.
90. Madura JA, Dibaise JK. Quick fix or long-term cure? Pros and cons of bariatric surgery. *F1000 Med Rep.* 2012;4:19.
91. American Society for Metabolic and Bariatric Surgery (ASMBS). Estimate of Bariatric Surgery Numbers, 2011–2015. Gainesville, FL: ASMBS; July 2016 [June 20, 2017]; Available at https://asmbs.org/resources/estimate-of-bariatric-surgery-numbers.
92. Brantley PJ, Waldo K, Matthews-ewald MR, et al. Why patients seek bariatric surgery: does insurance coverage matter? *Obes Surg.* 2014;24(6):961-4.
93. Kolotkin RL, Andersen JR. A systematic review of reviews: exploring the relationship between obesity, weight loss and health-related quality of life. *Clin Obes.* 2017;7(5):273-289.
94. Opozda M, Wittert G, Chur-Hansen A. Patients' reasons for and against undergoing Roux-en-Y gastric bypass, adjustable gastric banding, and vertical sleeve gastrectomy. *Surg Obes Relat Dis.* 2017;13(11):1887-1896.

95. Meguid MM, Glade MJ, Middleton FA. Weight regain after Roux-en-Y: a significant 20% complication related to PYY. *Nutrition.* 2008;24(9):832-42.
96. Cambi MP, Marchesini SD, Baretta GA. Post-bariatric surgery weight regain: evaluation of nutritional profile of candidate patients for endoscopic argon plasma coagulation. *Arq Bras Cir Dig.* 2015;28(1):40-3.
97. Svensson PA, Anveden Å, Romeo S, et al. Alcohol consumption and alcohol problems after bariatric surgery in the Swedish obese subjects study. *Obesity (Silver Spring).* 2013;21(12):2444-51.
98. King WC, Chen J-Y, et al. Prevalence of alcohol use disorders before and after bariatric surgery. *JAMA.* 2012;307(23):2516-2525.
99. Sjostrom L, Narbro K, et al. Effects of bariatric surgery on mortality in Swedish obese subjects. *N Engl J Med.* 2007; 357(8), 741-752.
100. Bariatric Surgery Source website: *https://www.bariatric-surgery-source.com.* Accessed March 5, 2019.
101. Sethi M, Chau E, Youn A, Jiang Y, Fielding G, Ren-Fielding C. Long-term outcomes after biliopancreatic diversion with and without duodenal switch: 2-, 5-, and 10-year data. *Surg Obes Relat Dis.* 2016;12(9):1697-1705.
102. Forbes R, Gasevic D, Watson EM, et al. Essential fatty acid plasma profiles following gastric bypass and adjusted gastric banding bariatric surgeries. *Obes Surg.* 2016;26(6):1237-46.
103. Westman EC. Personal communication, 2014.
104. Busetto L, Dicker D, Azran C, et al. Practical Recommendations of the Obesity Management Task Force of the European Association for the Study of Obesity for the Post-Bariatric Surgery Medical Management. *Obes Facts.* 2017;10(6):597-632.
105. Bast JH, Ahmed L, Engdahl R. Lipedema in patients after bariatric surgery. *Surg Obes Relat Dis.* 2016;12(5):1131-2.
106. Lipedema & KETO Way of Eating Facebook group: *https://www.facebook.com/groups/LipedemaKetoWOE/.*
107. Odom J, Zalesin KC, Washington TL, et al. Behavioral predictors of weight regain after bariatric surgery. *Obes Surg.* 2010;20(3):349-56.
108. García Botero A, García Wenninger M, Fernández Loaiza D. Complications after body contouring surgery in postbariatric patients. *Ann Plast Surg.* 2017;79(3):293-297.
109. Benatti F, Solis M, Artioli G, et al. Liposuction induces a compensatory increase of visceral fat which is effectively counteracted by physical activity: a randomized trial. *J Clin Endocrinol Metab.* 2012;97(7):2388-95.
110. Rapprich S, Dingler A, Podda M. Liposuction is an effective treatment for lipedema-results of a study with 25 patients. *J Dtsch Dermatol Ges.* 2011;9(1):33-40.
111. Wollina U, Graf A, Hanisch V. Acute pulmonary edema following liposuction due to heart failure and atypical pneumonia. *Wien Med Wochenschr.* 2015;165(9-10):189-94.
112. Peled AW, Kappos EA. Lipedema: diagnostic and management challenges. *Int J Womens Health.* 2016;8:389-95.
113. Fomin DA, McDaniel B, Crane J. The promising potential role of ketones in inflammatory dermatologic disease: a new frontier in treatment research. *J Dermatolog Treat.* 2017;28(6):484-487.
114. Hernandez TL, Kittelson JM, Law CK, et al. Fat redistribution following suction lipectomy: defense of body fat and patterns of restoration. *Obesity* (Silver Spring). 2011;19(7):1388-95.

115. Lee JY, Keane MG, Pereira S. Diagnosis and treatment of gallstone disease. *Practitioner*. 2015;259(1783):15-9, 2.
116. Bonfrate L, Wang DQ, Garruti G, Portincasa P. Obesity and the risk and prognosis of gallstone disease and pancreatitis. *Best Pract Res Clin Gastroenterol*. 2014;28(4):623-35.
117. Festi D, Colecchia A, Orsini M, et al. Gallbladder motility and gallstone formation in obese patients following very low calorie diets. Use it (fat) to lose it (well). *Int J Obes Relat Metab Disord*. 1998;22(6):592-600.
118. Gebhard RL, Prigge WF, Ansel HJ, et al. The role of gallbladder emptying in gallstone formation during diet-induced rapid weight loss. *Hepatology*. 1996;24(3):544-8.
119. Heshka S, Anderson JW, Atkinson RL, et al. Weight loss with self-help compared with a structured commercial program: a randomized trial. *JAMA*. 2003;289(14):1792-8.
120. Liem RK, Niloff PH. Prophylactic cholecystectomy with open gastric bypass operation. *Obes Surg* 2004;14:763–765.
121. Stokes CS, Gluud LL, Casper M, Lammert F. Ursodeoxycholic acid and diets higher in fat prevent gallbladder stones during weight loss: a meta-analysis of randomized controlled trials. *Clin Gastroenterol Hepatol*. 2014;12(7):1090-1100.e2.
122. Lengyel BI, Panizales MT, Steinberg J, Ashley SW, Tavakkoli A. Laparoscopic cholecystectomy: What is the price of conversion? *Surgery*. 2012;152(2):173-8.
123. Kraemer FB, Ginsberg HN. Gerald M. Reaven, MD: Demonstration of the central role of insulin resistance in type 2 diabetes and cardiovascular disease. *Diabetes Care*. 2014;37(5):1178-81.
124. Gami AS, Witt BJ, Howard DE, et al. Metabolic syndrome and risk of incident cardiovascular events and death: a systematic review and meta-analysis of longitudinal studies. *J Am Coll Cardiol*. 2007;49(4):403-14.
125. Aguilar M, Bhuket T, Torres S, Liu B, Wong RJ. Prevalence of the metabolic syndrome in the United States, 2003-2012. *JAMA*. 2015;313(19):1973-4.
126. Passare G, Viitanen M, Törring O, Winblad B, Fastbom J. Sodium and potassium disturbances in the elderly : prevalence and association with drug use. *Clin Drug Investig*. 2004;24(9):535-44.
127. Balci AK, Koksal O, Kose A, et al. General characteristics of patients with electrolyte imbalance admitted to emergency department. *World J Emerg Med*. 2013;4(2):113-6.
128. Sigler MH. The mechanism of the natriuresis of fasting. *J Clin Invest*. 1975;55(2):377-87.
129. DiNicolantonio J. *The Salt Fix, How the Experts Got It All Wrong--And Why Eating More Might Save Your Life*. Harmony; 2017. ISBN: 9780451496966.
130. Volek JS, Phinney SD. *The Art and Science of Low Carbohydrate Living: An Expert Guide to Making the Life-Saving Benefits of Carbohydrate Restriction Sustainable and Enjoyable*. Boca Raton: Beyond Obesity, LLC, 2011. ISBN: 9780983490708.
131. Casley-Smith JR. *Modern Treatment for Lymphoedema, Fifth Revised Edition*. The Lymphoedma Association of Australia, Inc., 1997, p 319. ISBN: 9780646316642.
132. Mente A, O'Donnell M, Rangarajan S, et al. Associations of urinary sodium excretion with cardiovascular events in individuals with and without hypertension: a pooled analysis of data from four studies. *Lancet*. 2016;388(10043):465-75.
133. Jantsch J, Schatz V, Friedrich D, et al. Cutaneous Na+ storage strengthens the antimicrobial barrier function of the skin and boosts macrophage-driven host defense. *Cell Metab*. 2015;21(3):493-501.
134. Crescenzi R, Marton A, Donahue PMC, et al. Tissue Sodium Content is Elevated

in the Skin and Subcutaneous Adipose Tissue in Women with Lipedema. *Obesity (Silver Spring)*. 2018;26(2):310-317.

135. Volek J, Phinney S. Virta Health blog. Available at *https://blog.virtahealth.com/sodium-nutritional-ketosis-keto-flu-adrenal-function/*

136. Coleman-Jensen A, Rabbitt MP, et al. Household food security in the United States in 2015. US Department of Agriculture, Economic Research Service. 2016. Available at *http://www.ers.usda.gov/media/2137657/err215_summary.pdf*. Accessed March 16, 2018.

137. Hales CM, Carroll MD, Fryar CD, Ogden CL. Prevalence of Obesity Among Adults and Youth: United States, 2015-2016. *NCHS Data Brief*. 2017;(288):1-8.

138. Ngaruiya C, Hayward A, Post L, Mowafi H. Obesity as a form of malnutrition: over-nutrition on the Uganda "malnutrition" agenda. *Pan Afr Med J*. 2017;28:49. Published 2017 Sep 20.

139. Coulthard MG. Oedema in kwashiorkor is caused by hypoalbuminaemia. *Paediatr Int Child Health*. 2015;35(2):83-9.

140. Braamskamp MJ, Dolman KM, Tabbers MM. Clinical practice. Protein-losing enteropathy in children. *Eur J Pediatr*. 2010;169(10):1179-85.

141. Pollan M. *In Defense of Food: An Eater's Manifesto*. New York, New York: Penguin Press; 2009. ISBN: 978-1594201455.

142. Martínez Steele E, Baraldi LG, Louzada ML, Moubarac JC, Mozaffarian D, Monteiro CA. Ultra-processed foods and added sugars in the US diet: evidence from a nationally representative cross-sectional study. *BMJ Open*. 2016;6(3):e009892.

143. Grover Z, Ee LC. Protein energy malnutrition. *Pediatric Clinics of North America*. 2009;56(5):1055-1068.

144. Mauron J, Antener I. Is the adult protein-energy malnutrition syndrome the same as that described in the infant? *Experientia Suppl*. 1983;44:298-338.

145. Ibrahim MK, Zambruni M, Melby CL, Melby PC. Impact of childhood malnutrition on host defense and infection. *Clin Microbiol Rev*. 2017;30(4):919-971.

146. Calder PC. The relationship between the fatty acid composition of immune cells and their function. *Prostaglandins Leukot Essent Fatty Acids*. 2008;79(3-5):101-8.

147. Astley S, Finglas P. *Reference Module in Food Science*. Elsevier, 2016.

148. Peumans WJ, Van Damme EJ. Lectins as plant defense proteins. *Plant Physiol*. 1995;109(2): 347-52.

149. Mudaliar S, Chang AR, Henry RR. Thiazolidinediones, peripheral edema, and type 2 diabetes: incidence, pathophysiology, and clinical implications. *Endocr Pract*. 2003;9(5):406-16.

150. Langsjoen PH, Langsjoen AM. Supplemental ubiquinol in patients with advanced congestive heart failure. *BioFactors*. 2008;32:119-128.

151. Honore PM, Jacobs R, Hendrickx I, et al. Statins and the Kidney: Friend or Foe? *Blood Purif*. 2017;43(1-3):91-96.

152. Morris DM, Jenkins GR. Preparing Physical and Occupational Therapists to Be Health Promotion Practitioners: A Call for Action. *Int J Environ Res Public Health*. 2018;15(2).

153. Institute of Medicine (US) Committee on Nutrition Services for Medicare Beneficiaries. (2000). The Role of Nutrition in Maintaining Health in the Nation's Elderly: Evaluating Coverage of Nutrition Services for the Medicare Population. Washington (DC): National Academies Press (US), 13, Providers of Nutrition Services. Available from: *https://www.ncbi.nlm.nih.gov/books/NBK225306/*.

154. DiMaria-Ghalili RA, Mirtallo JM, Tobin BW, Hark L, Van horn L, Palmer CA.

Challenges and opportunities for nutrition education and training in the health care professions: intraprofessional and interprofessional call to action. *Am J Clin Nutr.* 2014;99(5 Suppl):1184S-93S.
155. Lang J, James C, et al. The provision of weight management advice: An investigation into occupational therapy practice. *Australian Occupational Therapy Journal.* 2013;60:387-394.
156. Haracz K, Ryan S, Hazelton M, James C. Occupational therapy and obesity: an integrative literature review. *Aust Occup Ther J.* 2013;60(5):356-65.
157. American Physical Therapy Association (APTA). The Role of the Physical Therapist in Diet and Nutrition, HOD P06-15-22-17. June 3,2015. Available at http://www.apta.org/PatientCare/Nutrition. Accessed on April 15, 2018.
158. Butryn ML, Webb V, Wadden TA. Behavioral treatment of obesity. *Psychiatr Clin North Am.* 2011;34(4):841-59.
159. Sniehotta FF, Dombrowski SU, Avenell A, et al. Randomised controlled feasibility trial of an evidence-informed behavioural intervention for obese adults with additional risk factors. *PLoS ONE.* 2011;6(8):e23040.
160. Mallinson T, Fischer H, Rogers JC, Ehrlich-Jones L, Chang R. Human occupation for public health promotion: new directions for occupational therapy practice with persons with arthritis. *Am J Occup Ther.* 2009 Mar-Apr;63(2):220-6.
161. Gellert KS, Aubert RE, Mikami JS. Ke 'Ano Ola: Moloka'i's community-based healthy lifestyle modification program. *Am J Public Health.* 2010;100(5):779-83.
162. Digenio AG, Mancuso JP, Gerber RA, Dvorak RV. Comparison of methods for delivering a lifestyle modification program for obese patients: a randomized trial. *Ann Intern Med.* 2009;150(4):255-62.
163. Ash S, Reeves M, Bauer J, et al. A randomised control trial comparing lifestyle groups, individual counselling and written information in the management of weight and health outcomes over 12 months. *Int J Obes (Lond).* 2006;30(10):1557-64.
164. Wadden TA, Berkowitz RI, Womble LG, et al. Randomized trial of lifestyle modification and pharmacotherapy for obesity. *N Engl J Med.* 2005;353(20):2111-20.
165. Foster GD, Wyatt HR, Hill JO, et al. Weight and metabolic outcomes after 2 years on a low-carbohydrate versus low-fat diet: a randomized trial. *Ann Intern Med.* 2010;153(3):147-57.
166. Heshka S, Anderson JW, Atkinson RL, et al. Weight loss with self-help compared with a structured commercial program: a randomized trial. *JAMA.* 2003;289(14):1792-8.
167. Piller N. Links between BMI and the increasing incidence/prevalence of chronic oedema: What is our future? *J Lymphoedema.* 2016;11(1), 5-6.
168. Rippe JM, Crossley S, Ringer R. Obesity as a chronic disease: modern medical and lifestyle management. *J Am Diet Assoc.* 1998;98(10 Suppl 2):S9-15
169. Henderson E. Obesity in primary care: a qualitative synthesis of patient and practitioner perspectives on roles and responsibilities. *Br J Gen Pract.* 2015;65(633):e240-7.
170. Wicks A, Jamieson M. New ways for occupational scientists to tackle "wicked problems" impacting population health. *J Occup Sci.* 2014;21(1):1-5.
171. Weger Jr H, Bell CG, et al. The relative effectiveness of active listening in initial interactions, International Journal of Listening. 2014;28(1):13-31.
172. Johnson SS, Paiva AL, Cummins CO, et al. Transtheoretical model-based multiple behavior intervention for weight management: effectiveness on a population basis. *Prev Med.* 2008;46(3):238-46.

173. Miller WR, Rollnick S. *Motivational Interviewing, Second Edition: Preparing People for Change*. The Guilford Press; 1991. ISBN: 973-1-57230-563-2.
174. Carels RA, Darby L, Cacciapaglia HM, et al. Using motivational interviewing as a supplement to obesity treatment: a stepped-care approach. *Health Psychol*. 2007;26(3):369-74.
175. DiMarco ID, Klein DA, Clark VL, Wilson GT. The use of motivational interviewing techniques to enhance the efficacy of guided self-help behavioral weight loss treatment. *Eat Behav*. 2009;10(2):134-6.
176. Weiss J, Daniel T. Validation of the lymphedema life impact scale (LLIS): a condition-specific measurement tool for persons with lymphedema. *Lymphology*. 2015;48(3):128-38.
177. Neves PO, Andrade J, Monção H. Coronary artery calcium score: current status. *Radiol Bras*. 2017;50(3):182-189.
178. Ho KS, Tan CY, Mohd daud MA, Seow-choen F. Stopping or reducing dietary fiber intake reduces constipation and its associated symptoms. *World J Gastroenterol*. 2012;18(33):4593-6.
179. Shin JR, Ly SY. Dietary habits and factors related to lifestyles in constipated female students. *Kor J Comm Nutr*. 2003;8(5), 675-688.
180. Ramos CI, Andrade de Lima AF, Grilli DG, Cuppari L. The short-term effects of olive oil and flaxseed oil for the treatment of constipation in hemodialysis patients. *J Ren Nutr*. 2015; 25(1):50-6.
181. Harcombe Z, Baker JS, Cooper SM, et al. Evidence from randomised controlled trials did not support the introduction of dietary fat guidelines in 1977 and 1983: a systematic review and meta-analysis. *Open Heart*. 2015;2(1):e000196.
182. Davis W. *Wheat Belly: Lose the Wheat, Lose the Weight, and Find Your Path Back to Health*. New York, New York: Rodale, Inc., 2011. ISBN: 9781609611545.
183. Perlmutter D, Loberg K. *Grain Brain: The Surprising Truth About Wheat, Carbs, and Sugar—Your Brain's Silent Killers*. Little Brown and Company: 2013. ISBN: 978-0-316-23480-1.
184. de la Monte SM, Wands JR. Alzheimer's disease is type 3 diabetes-evidence reviewed. *J Diabetes Sci Technol*. 2008;2(6):1101-13.

# About the Author

Leslyn Keith, OTD, CLT-LANA, has a Clinical Doctorate in Occupational Therapy with an emphasis on lymphedema and obesity. She was certified as a Lymphedema Therapist in 2000 and became LANA-certified in 2001. Dr. Keith has started four lymphedema therapy programs in California including two in private practice.

In addition to treating lymphedema and other lymphatic disorders, she currently researches, consults, and lectures on lymphedema, lipedema, and obesity nationally. She is also an instructor for Klose Training.

Her professional memberships include the American Occupational Therapy Association, National Lymphedema Network, Lymphology Association of North America, Obesity Medicine Association, and International Society of Lymphology.

She can be contacted via email at leslynkeithot@gmail.com and more information about Dr. Keith can be found on her website at leslynkeith.com.

Made in United States
Cleveland, OH
26 April 2025

16434883R00079